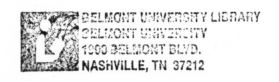

Address:

THE ESSENTIAL GUIDE TO THE INTERNET FOR HEALTH PROFESSIONALS

SYDNEY S. CHELLEN

There is a wealth of health information on the Internet. Today's students of health studies and all health care professionals must be able to use this valuable resource and extract from it what is most relevant and useful. In order for them to do this purposefully and skilfully, they need to have a thorough understanding of how the system works and have the ability to navigate their way around it with ease.

The Essential Guide to the Internet for Health Professionals is a superb photo-copiable resource for lecturers and a self-instructional guide for students. It shows students how to:

- get online;
- navigate the World Wide Web;
- find health information on the Internet;
- communicate with other health professionals;
- access free health and medical resources;
- publish on the web;
- use online help with health studies assignments;
- search for jobs.

Each unit contains easy-to-follow activities and photocopiable worksheets.

the essential guide to the

internet

For Health Professionals

Sydney S. Chellen is a Senior Lecturer in the Faculty of Nursing, Midwifery and Social Work, Canterbury Christ Church University College. He currently teaches Research and Information Technology to students on diploma, degree and other postgraduate programmes.

the essential guide to the

internet

Sydney S. Chellen

MA (KENT), BA (Ed.), PGCE (FE), RNT, RCNT, RMN, RN

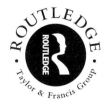

London and New York

First published 2000 by Routledge
11 New Fetter Lane, London EC4P 4EE

Simultaneously published in the USA and Canada
by Routledge
29 West 35th Street, New York, NY 10001

Reprinted 2002

Routledge is an imprint of the Taylor & Francis Group

Designed and typeset in Optima and Courier by Keystroke, Jacaranda Lodge, Wolverhampton
Printed and bound in Great Britain by St Edmundsbury Press Ltd, Bury St Edmunds, Suffolk

Disclaimer
Because the author has no control over the circumstances of use of this book, he cannot assume liability or responsibility for any consequential loss or damage, however caused, arising as a result of carrying out the activities in the book. The material is offered to the user on the basis of this understanding.

All the information in the book is believed to be correct at the time of writing. Whenever possible the author will try to assist with any queries.

PERMISSIONS AND CREDITS
All product and company names and ™ or ® trademarks of their respective owners.

Screenshots used with permission from appropriate copyright holders.

British Library Cataloguing in Publication Data
A catalogue record for this book is available from the British Library

Library of Congress Cataloguing in Publication Data
Chellen, Sydney S., 1945–
    The essential guide to the Internet for health professionals : an interactive beginner's handbook / Sydney S. Chellen.
        p. cm.
    Includes bibliographical references and index.
    1. Medicine—Computer network resources.   2. Internet (Computer network)
    3. Medical informatics.   I. Title: Internet.   II. Title.

R119.9.C48 2000
025.06'61—dc21

                                                                99–054706

ISBN 0–415–22747–X

contents

The Health Services are responsible for the delivery of skilled and high quality care to their patients and clients. Nowhere are these objectives more important than in the fields of nursing, radiography, occupational therapy, physiotherapy, health promotion, and social work. And one important quality standard to be applied to the work in health studies and healthcare practice is that it is based on the use of the best information and best practice. The Internet is a subject in which many people are, let's face it, blissful innocents. I would urge you to take the Internet seriously and find out what is most relevant and useful – *The Essential Guide to the Internet* is a practical means towards that end.

This stimulating book sets out with clarity the framework provided by the Internet and examines in helpful detail how to use those parts of cyberspace that provide particularly relevant evidence – how to access the net, the webs, e-mail, Discussion Groups, Gateways to Health Resources, Jobsearch, and Publishing. It's a how-to book to get you going and save you time, with 17 worksheet activities (plus more on the net), illustrations, explanations, questions and answers, complete with many interesting and pertinent web sites.

Professor Bill Lemmer
Director, Centre for Health Services Research and
Head of Mental Health and Learning Disabilities
Canterbury Christ Church University College.
Founding Editor, *Journal of Psychiatric and Mental Health Nursing*
e-mail: w.e.lemmer@cant.ac.uk

As a student of health studies following a programme in higher education, you will be required to seek relevant information to deliver seminars and write lengthy academic essays. In the past, you would have needed to rely almost exclusively on the resources that are physically on the college campus to acquire this information. The **Internet** has changed all this. It has revolutionised the way students, like you, can enhance their programmes of study. The net has extended the learning resources to colleges, organisations and health experts around the globe, making it unnecessary for you to rely solely on your college library, your college lecturers or even purchasing expensive reference books.

The Internet is a gigantic computer network and you will be surprised how much health information you can uncover (eg, new drugs, online journals, medical schools, clinical guidelines, consumer health information and so on). It also offers you the opportunity to share your ideas with other disciplines and empower yourself. Therefore, it is not surprising that there has been an explosion of interest in the *Internet* since it hit the headlines in a big way in 1994. 'Surfing the net', the 'World Wide Web', 'Information Superhighway' and 'Cyberspace' are all colourful terms that are used to refer to the Internet. Millions of people use it every day, and the number is growing all the time. If you have the appropriate computer system at home, you can even access resources at your college/university (or elsewhere), and obtain limitless information cheaply and quickly.

Despite the mystique surrounding the net, virtually anyone can master the skills necessary to access it. Even if you are new to computers, once you have familiarised yourself with the basic procedures and concepts of using a PC (personal computer) in a **Windows** environment, you too will find it quite easy to use the Internet's many facilities purposefully.

Just take a quick look through the book, and you will see that it has been written for beginners like you. You will also notice that this is not just a book that talks about the Internet and its many wonders: it is a workbook that expects you to practise the skills as you go along. The book has been written in that form because I firmly believe that the only sure way of developing any skill, including Information Technology skills, is to practise. If this is what you feel you require, then this is the book for you.

Information Technology skills are quite complex. Nevertheless, an attempt has been made to split the task into a number of neat 'units' covering different aspects but, to avoid repetition, you will find frequent reference to work covered in earlier units/worksheets in the book. Wherever references have been made to past units or worksheets, look quickly back to the relevant section to remind yourself of what has been covered.

The **Internet** can be defined as a system that lets thousands of computers all over the world talk to each other.

Windows can be described as a collection of programs, or suite of programs, written for personal computers and published by Microsoft. It is sometimes referred to as a GUI (graphical user interface). There are three common versions around: Windows 3.1, Windows95 and Windows98, the third one being the most recent and most sophisticated, pending the arrival of yet another version called Windows 2000.

NOTE

As you work through this book you will come across the cue: activity . . . Worksheets to support certain activities are included. They are an integral part of the work of this book. So follow the instructions given. When you have completed each activity, return to the main text.

> **Broadly speaking, software refers to the programs which provide the driving force of all computing systems. There are two types: operating systems software and applications software.**

It should be appreciated that the **software** for using the many facilities on the net may vary from college to college and is in a constant state of change. For the purpose of illustrations and activities, I have chosen the network set-up and software available in the Canterbury Christ Church University College as this is where I am currently working. Even if the set-up and software available in your college or on your home system differ somewhat, you should still be able to benefit from the information in this book and carry out most of the activities set with minimum difficulty. I say this with great confidence as I too have a different set-up at home.

Your overall learning objective is therefore that when you have finished working through this book, you will have met the many inhabitants of the Internet, and will be able to surf the net and use many of its features with a high degree of understanding, competency and satisfaction.

Sydney S. Chellen
Senior Lecturer (Nursing Studies)
Canterbury Christ Church University College
e-mail: s.s.chellen@cant.ac.uk

30 January 1999

acknowledgements

I would like formally to acknowledge the support and advice of Karen E. Worden, Subject Librarian at Canterbury Christ Church University College, with the preparation of Unit 4 and related Worksheets.

I would also like to thank the following reviewers who critiqued the entire manuscript and offered excellent feedback, suggestions and support.

- Mooi Standing, Senior Lecturer: Nursing, Canterbury Christ Church University College
- Eddie Newall, Lecturer: Training and Development, Canterbury Christ Church University College
- Dr Sylvia Prosser, Principal Lecturer: Nursing, Canterbury Christ Church University College
- Professor W.E. Lemmer, Director: Centre for Health Services Research and Head of Mental Health and Learning Disabilities, Canterbury Christ Church University College. Also founding editor: *Journal of Psychiatric and Mental Health Nursing*
- Keith Jones, Hon. Research Fellow: Centre for Health Services Studies, University of Kent at Canterbury and Network Leader for LASERNET. Formerly Nursing Officer (Examinations Research), English National Board for Nursing, Midwifery and Health Visiting
- Patricia Chellen, School Teacher and Literacy Co-ordinator for Key Stage 2, Napier Primary School
- Students on the B.Sc. Nursing programme
- 1st-year students on the OT programme
- Radiography students on the M.Sc. programme
- Student nurses on Research modules
- Student nurses on the EN Conversion programme.
- Maurice V. Chellen, Law Student, Brunel University.

Dedicated to all the students who put this book to use

who should use this book?

The Essential Guide to the Internet is written for students following a course in health studies in a college of higher education. Anyone falling in the following categories should find it helpful:

- students following a Diploma in Nursing Studies (P2K);
- trainee midwives, health visitors, RNs converting to diploma;
- clinicians following a Bachelor or Master's programme or a path to the Higher Award in nursing, midwifery and health visiting;
- medical students (doctors – in particular junior doctors and GPs);
- members of the professions allied to medicine, eg trainee occupational therapists, physiotherapists, radiographers, speech therapists, dieticians, pharmacists, paramedics and so on; and
- those caring professionals who have picked up some cyberspace skills on an ad hoc basis, eg, Nurse Lecturers, Clinical Managers, etc.

how is this book structured?

The Essential Guide to the Internet is split into nine distinct yet related learning units. It includes the following features:

- **Self-selection of topics/concepts** – Each Unit is preceded with a picklist. Users are invited to select those items which interest them and they are then guided on how to proceed. This picklist provides a means of finding specific answers quickly and easily.

- **Suggested activities** – to help users develop specific skills.

- **Appendices** – containing the user agreement, UK service providers, country codes, error messages, glossary and references.

- **Glossary of terms** – A full list of essential terms for quick reference.

- **Recommended reading list** – In Appendix 6 users will find a carefully selected reading list for further knowledge development.

icons used

Additional textual information has been included in boxes. Four types of boxes have been used, and they appear throughout the book. Each type of box has been assigned a distinguishing icon to inform the reader of the type of information being read. They are as follows:

WARNING!

In this box the users will find information to warn them of possible dangers when carrying out certain procedures, or making a decision.

HOW?

In this box users will find information that will guide them to achieve specific objectives.

TECHNO TALK

In this box users will find an explanation of important concepts/technical terms that they might encounter when dealing with a part-icular area of the Internet.

NOTE

In this box users will find additional information to clarify a point or information that they might need at a later stage.

conventions used

For clarity, different type styles and keyboard conventions have also been used as shown below:

CONVENTION	MEANING
Bold face type	▶ Indicates an Internet, e-mail or newsgroup address or part of an address. ▶ Means text that you may need to type into the computer (input text should be typed as they appear).
Bold italic	▶ Indicates text you will type but I don't know exactly what it will be eg, a ***keyword***. ▶ Means text you would click on.
<u>**Bold-underline**</u>	Indicates a new computer word or expression being encountered.
Plain italic	Means a computer word or expression that has been previously defined and for quick reference can be found in the Glossary of terms at the end of the book.
ENTER (↵)	This means press the ENTER key on your keyboard. N.B. This key might be labelled 'RETURN' or simply have a symbol as shown in brackets here: (↵)

The Essential Guide to the Internet is self-paced and provides an individualised, interactive learning package. Users can read it from cover to cover if they so wish, but they don't have to. They will find that they can dip into any unit or section and learn something. The cross-references adopted in this book should lead/tempt them to other units/sections of the book. When carrying out the activities, it is important that users follow the instructions and apply some common sense. For example, if they find that after having carried out an instruction they do not get the expected result, they should backtrack and try again as they might have done something wrong.

some assumptions

It is assumed that the user will have some knowledge of computers and some understanding of Windows ie, how to switch on the computer, load Windows and use the mouse. Also that the user will be holding the mouse with the right hand. For information in the areas mentioned above, please see a copy of this book: Chellen, S.S.(1995) *Information Technology for the Caring Professions – A User's Handbook.* London: Cassell plc.

what will you achieve?

Each of the Units in *The Essential Guide to the Internet* will help you to develop your understanding of the Internet with opportunities to explore some of its inhabitants eg, Gophers, search engines, directories. To give you a feel for the book as a whole, the next page lists the most important learning objectives of each Unit.

UNIT	THIS UNIT WILL HELP YOU TO:
1 **Health and the net – an overview**	Examine the services available on the net and their benefits to students following a course in health studies in a college of higher education.
2 **Getting online**	Identify the process for getting online on the college computer network. Essential information is included for those of you who want to get on the net at home. This section contains four activities with worksheets to guide you.
3 **The World Wide Web**	Identify some important features of a browser and how to use it to explore the web. In this section you will find a selected list of UK and Foreign Internet sites applicable to Nursing and Allied professions. These sites are organised under thirteen distinct headings as follows:
	▶ Organisations, Associations and UK Statutory Bodies
	▶ Adult Nursing and Medicine
	▶ Alternative Medicine
	▶ General Health Information
	▶ Mental Health Nursing, Psychiatry and Learning Disabilities
	▶ Midwifery and Health Visiting
	▶ Paediatric Nursing and Medicine
	▶ Paramedical
	▶ Healthcare Research
	▶ Journals for Health Professions
	▶ Libraries and Free Health Databases
	▶ Electronic Publication and Citation
	▶ Quality of Public Services
4 **Finding health information on the Internet**	Familarise yourself with some of the net's inhabitants. Here you will find ten guided activities to help you explore specific databases using effective search strategies to find health information for your projects.
5 **Communicating with other health carers by e-mail**	Understand the basics of e-mail and develop skills of using a popular e-mail program. It includes information on e-mail conventions, e-mail overload and other related issues. In this section there are five activities with worksheets.
6 **Joining health discussion groups andmailing lists, starting IRC and VON**	Uncover some interesting health newsgroups and mailing lists where you can read messages on a variety of health topics and participate in online discussions, including real-time conferencing. It will also help you to examine software you need to access news (both at home or at your institution) and discuss relevant issues. Included here are four activities supported with worksheets.
7 **Gateway to free health and medical resources**	Experience using additional tools to make effective use of your net browser. There are four activities supported with worksheets giving you step-by-step instructions.
8 **Publishing on the web**	Develop an understanding of the design of a web page, and get started in creating a simple web page. There are two activities with worksheets.
9 **Online help with your health studies and jobs search**	Locate study tools, evaluate material available on the web, cite electronic sources correctly and use the services on the net to find a job.

health and the net – an overview

1

"The development of information processing and retrieval skills, with an ability to operate a computer and produce effective results in letters, documents, and reports, and educational materials, are now very important . . . for ourselves, our colleagues, our students." Ballard (1996)[1]

Senior Lecturer
School of Nursing and Midwifery,
University of Wolverhampton

Many healthcare students around the world are making it their business to learn how to surf the net because they have realised the wealth of health information it contains, and the opportunity it offers them to share ideas with other students and healthcare professionals around the world.

The volume of information available via the Internet is huge. Everything that may be of interest to you is scattered around the world on different computers. Collectively these computers make up the Internet. Here is a quick outline of the most popular services on offer that should get you interested:

- **World Wide Web** – which, among other things, contains a wealth of health information
- Searchable, browsable health and medical **databases**
- **E-mail** for two-way world wide communication
- **Newsgroups**: a discussion platform of topical health issues
- **Mailing lists** for keeping up to date in your specialist area
- **Internet Relay Chat** for distance learning
- **Voice on the net (VON)** for live communication
- **FTP** for looking inside distant computers
- **Archie** for copying files from distant computers
- **Gopher** as an alternative to the web
- **Telnet** to connect your home computer to others on the net
- Easy **publishing** on the web
- **Online help** to assist you eg with your study and jobsearch

1.1 the world wide web

(Also referred to as WWW or the web) is the graphical, multimedia portion of the Internet and is one of the most immediate, easy to use services on the net. It links all the **web pages** together. Thus, a page you're viewing from a computer in Canterbury may lead you to a page in New York, Ottawa, or Sydney with just one click of the mouse. You will find many Colleges, Universities, Libraries, and Health Institutions, including individual users and others with their own pages (called the homepage). You will be able to read material on almost any topic or any branch of healthcare. For example, if you have an interest in mental health you can pay a visit to the Mental HealthNet for information on interactive discussion groups, mental health administration tips, popular articles, self-help resources, tools and information for clinicians. Likewise, if you were interested in Adult or Childcare or Learning Disability you would find appropriate sites. As Howson (1997)[2] puts it:

> [Almost] whatever you need to know you will find a site to answer your question.

(A selected list of UK and Foreign web sites applicable to nursing and allied professions is given in Unit 3.) Should you require extra help with your studies, you will find interactive web-based tutorials, which you can explore at your own pace and when it suits you. You will also be able to access some Computer Assisted Learning materials and read up-to-date electronic health journals on a variety of health disciplines (*See Units 3 & 4*).

> **TECHNOTALK**
> To view different files on the web, you use web browsing software such as NetScape Navigator or Internet Explorer. Each file (or location) is called a <u>web page.</u>

1.2 databases

A range of commercial databases, increasingly with full-text services, is being delivered via the Internet. One of the leading electronic information retrieval services is Ovid Technologies Inc. The Ovid-Biomed service provides 'a fully functional, low cost, Medline service' to HE and FE institutions and NHS organisations. The service provides access to important databases, namely: Medline,

Cinahl, Cancerlit, Core Biomedical Collection, Ovid Biomedical Collection II, III, IV, Mental Health Collection and Nursing Collection. (The 'Collections' are smaller specialised databases put together by Ovid containing the electronic full text version of up to 20 relevant journals.)

The Ovid-Biomed Nursing Collection offers you the ability to search the database and link from the citation to the full text and print the complete article off to take away. It provides access to the following journals from 1995 onwards and is updated on a monthly basis:

- *Advances in Nursing Science*
- *American Journal of Infection Control*
- *AORN Journal*
- *Dermatology Nursing*
- *Heart and Lung*
- *Image: Journal of Nursing Scholarship*
- *Journal of Advanced Nursing*
- *Journal of Clinical Nursing*
- *Journal of Emergency Nursing*
- *Nurse Researcher*
- *Nursing Health Care*
- *Nursing Management (RCN Publishing)*
- *Nursing Standard*
- *RN*

NOTE

EBMR encompasses two major sources of evidence-based medicine material, the Cochrane Database of Systematic Reviews and Best Evidence.

You will also find that the Ovid-Biomed service has recently included Evidence Based Medicine Reviews (EBMR). This is a useful addition. You can perform a search using medline and retrieve additional information from an EBMR article.

These databases will help you to complete your course assignments. You will be able to interrogate these databases from the comfort of your home or your college computer lab.

It is, however, important to bear in mind that most institutions and organisations – based on the needs of their users and financial constraints – would have selected various combinations of Internet databases to subscribe to. So don't expect to be able to have access to all available electronic databases at your college, university computing laboratory or from your home system (*See Unit 4, Section 4.3*).

1.3 electronic mail (e-mail)

The Internet is a popular communications system that will be around for a long time to come. It brings together the best aspects of Postal mail, the telephone, the fax machine, the public/college library, and the newspaper while improving on their worst features. For example, its e-mail service provides you with an easier, cheaper and faster method of keeping in touch. You can use it to collaborate on common projects with healthcare students in places like America and Russia; or simply exchange personal messages with other healthcare colleagues, friends or relatives at other networked sites almost anywhere in the world – without the need to use paper, pen, envelope, stamp and post box. By drafting and sending e-mail to foreign healthcare students you will be able to increase your range of communication skills and extend your use of language. Although most e-mail messages are just ordinary text, you can attach almost any type of computer file you want to send along with it (such as a spreadsheet, word-processing document or even a picture), and encrypt the message so that no one except the intended recipient will be able to read it. When working in the community you will be able to quickly and efficiently transmit files and data 'back to base' or to other healthcare professionals from a portable or notebook computer, whilst on the move. By sharing information in this way you will help to enhance the quality, responsiveness, targeting and efficiency of healthcare in the NHS (*See Unit 5*).

1.4 newsgroups

These are discussion groups and each focus on one particular subject. The discussion itself takes place through a form of e-mail, but the major difference is that messages are passed around the whole group to read, and add to. There are hundreds of health groups you can join, such as nursing, midwifery, medical informatics, pharmacy, radiology and many more. If you like sharing your views with other Healthcare students or Health Professionals, you will find the Usenet newsgroup irresistible. It provides a forum for discussion of issues related to a wide range of specialist subjects. Here you will be able to engage around the clock in group discussions, exchange information and ideas with other health professionals all over the world and seek information from them. This is a great and fun way to test your thoughts on particular health issues (*See Unit 6, Section 6.1*).

1.5 mailing lists

This provides yet another way of keeping in touch with people who share your interest. The mailing list is a special kind of e-mail address that re-mails all incoming mail to a list of subscribers on the mailing list. Mailing lists differ from newsgroups in that a separate copy of the mailing list message is e-mailed to each recipient on the list. Each mailing list has a specific topic, so all you need to do is to subscribe to the ones that interest you (*See Unit 6, Section 6.2*).

1.6 internet relay chat (irc)

This is a novel, but unfortunately expensive way to communicate in 'real-time-typing'. Nevertheless, here you can hold conversations with one or more health professionals by typing messages back and forth that instantly appear on the screens of everyone involved (*See Unit 6, Section 6.3*).

1.7 voice on the net (von)

If your computer has a soundcard, and a microphone plugged into it, you can talk to anyone in the world just as you do with a telephone (provided they are online and have a soundcard and microphone too). Since your Internet call will be a local call, you may be able to hold conversations at a cheaper rate than using a telephone. In the not too distant future you will be able to access tutors over a two-way real-time video link between the college and clinical areas (*See Unit 6, Section 6.4*).

1.8 file transfer protocol (ftp)

NOTE

FTP is one of many protocols used to copy files from one computer to another on the Internet. Also used are terms like 'an FTP site' (a site that lets you grab files from it using this protocol).

The collections of computers that make up the Internet hold a combined library of millions of files. The FTP system lets you look inside directories on some of these computers and copy files straight to your hard disk just as if you were copying files between directories on your own computer system (*See Unit 7, Section 7.1*).

1.9 archie

Copying files from a distant computer to your own using FTP is quite simple, but first you have got to track down the file you want. If the file exists, Archie will help you to find it in seconds. All you will need to do is to enter the name of the file (or part of it) into a program that can search through indexes of files on computers on FTP sites (*See Unit 7, Section 7.2*).

1.10 gopher

If you are happy with the World Wide Web you may not be at all keen on Gopher. Nevertheless, Gopher is an older Internet filing system. It is menu-driven and offers an alternative way of searching, retrieving and reading materials from local and remote sites on the Internet. Although, since the arrival of the World Wide Web, Gopher's popularity has been on the decline – leaving a reduced number of links to Gopher sites – you should still find many useful documents stored on Gopher servers (*See Unit 7, Section 7.3*).

1.11 telnet

Telnet will let you connect from your home computer to your college computer across the Internet and use it as if you were directly connected to that computer. This can be quite useful if, for example, you need to search your college/university library catalogues for available books (*See Unit 7, Section 7.4*).

1.12 publishing on the net

Anyone can become an author on the Internet. You will be able to use the web to publish articles or results of a research project you have completed. You may even be interested in launching your own newsletter or web page (*See Unit 8*).

1.13 online help with your health studies and job search

<u>Online</u> classes are slowly appearing. At some web sites you will find information about examinations, tips for success, summaries for syllabuses and so on. You will also find useful web sites to help find a job in the healthcare profession (*See Unit 9*).

There are many more things to do on the net that makes it so compelling to "surf". In fact the Internet is the place to learn more about the Internet.

In this book I will tell you step-by-step how to get online using your home or college computer, how to find your way around and how to use most of the services mentioned above. I will show you how to use literature searching and evaluation strategies to access the information you need for your course assignments from Internet databases. I will also show you how to use the net to locate and correspond via e-mail with experts in your field, and to join chat groups plus more.

> **TECHNO TALK**
> <u>Online</u> is a synonym for 'connected'. Anything connected to your computer and ready for action can be said to be online. In *Internet* terms it means that you have successfully dialled in to your service provider's computer and are now connected to the net. The opposite term is *offline*.

There is a wealth of health information on the net. As a whole it has many users, but the World Wide Web is the most popular and e-mail is growing in use all the time. There are many different ways of getting the information, some more expensive than others, but once you have the knowledge to use them, you can choose the best way for you.

2

"The hardest thing for me was getting started, but once I was hooked-up I just could not get off. I have splashed out on a computer system, and I go online every evening, checking my e-mail box and participating in newsgroups."

Student on Project 2000
Canterbury Christ Church University College, Kent

TECHNOTALK

Account is a term used in computer science to describe a Record-keeping arrangement employed by a System Manager at a College, University or health organisation, and a Vendor of an online service. It helps Vendors to identify their subscribers, for example, for billing. System Managers of multi-user systems use it to identify their users for administration and security purposes. A personal computing account is rather like your bank account. This has a Password (ie, a secret code used to keep things private) that 'only' you know, together with an account name (Username) that identifies you.

Username is a unique name you are assigned by a service that enables you to connect to it and identify yourself, demonstrating that you are entitled to access it.

This is another way of saying getting connected to the Internet. There are different ways to get online, but as a healthcare student registered for any part time or full time course at a university or college where computing facilities with Internet connection are in place, all you will need to start surfing the net is an **account**. Then, as long as you remain a student at that college and you comply with your user agreement (See **Appendix 1**) you will enjoy unlimited free access. However, if you would like to surf the net in the comfort of your home you will need the appropriate bits and pieces. This Unit will help you to identify the process of getting online at the college. You will also find essential information on how to get on the net at home.

checklist

Below is a checklist of what you can expect to find out in this Unit. Read through the statements then tick (✓) the items about which you would like to know more.

I would like to find out more about:

Please turn over the page and read through the topics you have ticked

You cannot get a *Username* and *Password* until an account has been set up for you. Once this has been done, you will be able to use your allocated Username and Password to access the computer and get on the Net and do many of the things outlined in unit one.

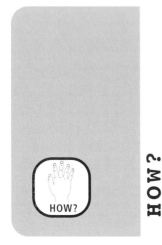

HOW?

How to obtain a college computing account?

Once you are a fully registered student on a course of study, you will normally be given information about the computing facilities available, where you will find them, how to obtain a personal computing account, what to do should you need technical help, and so on. If this has not happened in your case, you should contact your personal tutor and/or Computing Services Department and someone will set up an account for you. In some colleges you will find a system of self-registration is available. If this is the case, you will be able to use virtually any PC in the computing laboratories or an Open Access Area for this purpose. The self-registration procedure is usually quite simple. After registration you usually will need to wait 24 hours before you can log on the network.

2.1.1 ten key points for protecting your password

As a healthcare student, at the end of your course, you will most probably join a hospital Trust, where, as part of your daily work, you are going to be using a computer system containing data about patients. It is, therefore, vital that right from the start, you get into the good habit of taking extra care of your *Username* and *Password*. You can start practising good habits during your period in college/university. Here are ten key points to help you on your way:

1. Never type your Password in front of another person where (s)he can see the keys you press.
2. Never use swear words because they are easier to guess.
3. Never use the following as a Password: your Username, the name of the computer you are logged into, the name of your department, or words such as "PASSWORDS" or "SECRET", because they are words that immediately come to everyone's mind.
4. Never use any word, name or number that has an obvious association with you personally, such as your own name or nickname, name of your spouse, partner, boyfriend, girlfriend, name of your child or pet, your own date of birth or that of a member of your family, your car registration number, your telephone number, or name of the town in which you live.
5. Never choose a plain English word or a personal name as a Password – because a "**hacker**" can write a program that runs through a computerised dictionary trying every word as a Password.

Hacker is a term normally used to describe a skilled programmer who invades systems and ferrets out information on individual computer access codes through a process of trial and error

TECHNO TALK

⑥ Always change your Password on a regular basis – normally the computer system will force you to change it periodically.

⑦ Always change your Password if you suspect that it may have been discovered by someone else.

⑧ Always keep your Username and Password secret – avoid writing it down.

⑨ Always make sure you remember your Password.

⑩ Always choose a Password that will lodge in your mind so that you will not need to write it down. For example, use unusual words with at least six characters long combining letters and numbers such as 12blue.

2.1.2 choosing and remembering a password

When choosing a password you should always make sure that it will be easy for you to remember, and difficult for others to guess. Here are a few suggestions for you to consider:

▷ Select the first letter of each word of your favourite proverb, catchphrase or song eg, **IHSSIWF** (I Have Started So I Will Finish); **YSFT** (Your Starter For Ten).

▷ Select two colours and join them together eg, **redblue**

▷ Select a significant year and spell some of the digits eg, **10SIXTY6** or **TEN66**

▷ Select an English word you use a lot and add a 2-digit number before or after it eg, **18LOVE** or **LOVE18** (the number could be the first or last two numbers of your telephone or year of birth).

▷ Select two words which are the opposite of each other eg **YESNO**

▷ If you have been allocated a Password that you can't change, you can make it easier to remember by creating a mnemonic. For example, if your Password is **wkj11** you could remember it as **Willie King John the eleventh**.

2.2 getting started with the college computing system

Once an account has been set up and you are in possession of a working Username and Password, you are ready to log on to the Internet. All you now need to do is to take yourself to a computer lab and sit down in front of a Windows NT workstation. Before doing the next activity, here are a few words about the rules that you must obey, at all times, when using college computing facilities.

2.2.1 regulations governing college computing facilities

All colleges, universities and Trust hospitals that provide computing facilities will have "Regulations" governing their use. The full text of these regulations will have been issued to you or may simply be displayed in computing laboratories and perhaps in certain other places. It is usually deemed to be your responsibility to read these regulations and to ensure that you comply with them. Failure to adhere to the rules could lead to your being banned from using the network and disciplinary action taken against you. By way of example, I have included in **Appendix 1**, a typical User agreement that you can expect from colleges, universities, when you register to use computing facilities.

activity 2.1 LOGGING ON TO YOUR COLLEGE COMPUTER SYSTEM

Get to a computer laboratory in your college and sit yourself in front of a Windows NT workstation. Now, using your allocated Username and Password, log ON to the system.

WARNING!

```
If you have difficulty logging ON, you should seek help from the Helpdesk at
your institutions, otherwise you will not be able to use your college system
to get on the Net, nor will you be able to carry out the other activities in
this book.
```

Once you have logged ON successfully, familiarise yourself with the Windows environment including making sure you know how to log OFF properly.

When you have completed the activity return to this page and read on

2.3 getting started with a computing system at home

There will be times when you would wish you can work on your health projects or other course assignments and do your literature search while sitting in the comfort of your home. You now can and it need not cost you an arm and a leg. As mentioned already, to get *online* at home you first need a few bits and pieces. You may already have a few of them. Carry out Activity 2.2 below, this inventory will help you determine your current position.

Here is a list of what you will need to start surfing the net at home. Use this checklist to tick (✓) your requirements:

checklist:

- ⊙ a computer
- ⊙ a **modem** to use with your computer
- ⊙ a telephone line to connect your modem
- ⊙ communication software to drive your modem
- ⊙ membership of a **service provider** to get on the Internet
- ⊙ an electronic name and address. (This will be issued to you by the service provider, when you join a service)
- ⊙ the electronic name and address of the person you are attempting to communicate with.

Below you will find some information about each of the bits on the checklist above that you might find useful.

> A **modem** is a device that converts data back and forth between the format recognised by computers and the format needed to send it down the telephone line.
>
> **Service Provider** is a general term for a company that gives you access to the Internet by letting you dial in to its computer. This may be an Internet service provider (ISP) or an online service provider (IOP). For additional information see Section 2.3.5

2.3.1 which computer?

There are several families of computers on the market. Almost anyone with a computer will be up to the task. However, the healthcare Trusts and most Colleges/Universities are using **IBM** or IBM compatible computers. It will therefore make good sense to opt for one of those. There is also the question of whether you should opt for a **laptop** or **desktop**. Here are a few suggestions that you might find useful when making a decision to purchase a computer.

▶ **Laptop vs desktop** – Unless you plan to travel a lot with your computer, you will be better off with a desktop. Purely and simply because you will pay less for the same performance.

▶ **Speed** – Faster models are coming out almost every year. The Pentium range of computers is quite fast. These are fitted with different types of Pentium chips. Some Pentium chips are faster than others. The speed at which a chip can process information is measured in megahertz (MHz). The slowest Pentium chip works at 60Mhz and the fastest (at the time of writing) is 850Mhz. Although you do not need the fastest chip in your computer to surf the Net, I can assure you, the faster the computer, the more likely you are to enjoy your online search, and the longer it is likely to serve you. So go for the newest and fastest model you can afford.

▶ **Windows** – Windows 95 has built-in support for Internet connections that make all the setting-up easy. Windows 98 makes connections even easier as it includes a Microsoft's own browser: Internet Explorer. Looming on the horizon is Windows 2000.

> **IBM (Short for International Business Machines)** is an American computer manufacturer, with headquarters in Armonk, New York. The company is a major supplier of information-processing products in the United States and around the world. Its products are used in a wide variety of industries, including business, government, science, defence, education, medicine, and space exploration.
>
> A **Laptop** is a type of computer light enough for you to use while resting it on your lap and because it weighs around 9 to 12 pounds it can also be carried around. A **Desktop** computer as the name suggests is kept on top of a desk or any suitable hard work surface.

- **RAM** – When surfing the Net, there are times when your computer will need to be able to temporarily remember lots of information at once. The amount of random access memory (**RAM**) available in your computer will matter. The more RAM memory there is, the more information your computer will be able to remember simultaneously. RAM, which is measured in megabytes (MB, where 1024 kilobytes [KB] equals 1 MB), is limited by the amount that your machine can support and you can afford. As programs are getting bigger, 32MB of RAM is becoming the absolute minimum in a new machine. However, you should consider at least 64MB or even 128MB.

- **Hard disk** – This provides a place to store software programs along with any information that you may have in RAM and want to keep. The hard disk is a vital piece of hardware, as you will need to install a few new programs to get on the Net. You will also require storage space if you plan to download some of the free software available on the Net. Hard disks come in two main varieties: 'IDE' (Intelligent Drive Electronics) and 'SCSI' (Small Computer System Interface). Hard disks tend to fill more quickly than you would think, especially after you've been online for a while and have accumulated an impressive healthcare library of your own. Most new desktop machines come with a minimum of 4.5 gigabytes (GB) of hard disk space, more than enough for Internet use. If you plan to **download** a lot of images, get one with 6.5 GB hard drive or larger. A gigabyte is about 1,000 megabytes.

- **Sound card** – If you would like to use Voice (see section 6.4) and hear musical offerings on the Net, then you'll need a sound card. There are various types. An example is a 32-bit AWE sound card by Creative Labs.

- **Monitor** (VDU – Video Display Unit) – This is a critical component of your computer system. As you will be staring at the monitor for long hours when surfing the Net, you must get a good quality monitor. There are important standards to look for. The most important are: Resolution, Size, **Refresh Rate**, Memory, Bus type, Knobs and Swivels. Activity 2.3 will help you identify the quality of the monitor you have or are planning to have.

- **Keyboard and mouse/track balls** – Keyboards have a fairly standard layout, but they do differ in terms of ergonomics and feel. There are many types of mouse, and each one feels different. The keyboard and the mouse are the two items you will use to give instructions to the computer. When surfing the Net you will probably use the mouse most. So get yourself a good one, that you feel comfortable with. If you have difficulty using a mouse, you may want to consider a Track ball instead. This is like an upside-down mouse with the roller ball exposed. To make a movement, you roll the ball itself.

- **Printer** – Strictly speaking you do not need a printer to surf the Net. But if while trawling the net you find useful information to complete your health project or other assignments, to print out your find you will need a printer.

As can be expected a variety of printers exist, but really there are principally three types to choose from. Here they are in order of increasing quality and cost: **dot matrix**, **inkjet** and **Laser**. For most work you should find inkjet quite adequate. Here is a checklist of other factors to consider:

- speed
- colour or black and white output
- running cost
- noise level
- paper handling
- size

To enjoy the World Wide Web you will be happiest with a display unit that has the following spec or better. Use this checklist and tick (✓) the specification (spec) of the monitor you have or are planning to buy.

checklist:

- A VGA monitor which can display 256 colours with a resolution of 800x600 or an SVGA 256-colour monitor with a resolution of 1024x768
- 17 inch screen
- with a screen refresh rate of 70Hz
- 2MB video card
- VESA (Video Electronics Standards Association) or PCI (Peripheral Component Interconnect) bus
- non-interlaced scanning
- has touch-buttons or knobs to adjust settings such as brightness, contrast etc., and
- has a stand that swivels so that you can adjust it

2.3.2 which modem?

Your *modem* is one of the key links between your computer and your Internet service provider. The other link is your telephone line. Two of the most important features to look for when choosing a modem are: speed and compatibility. The faster the modem, the quicker it will move information from one end to the other, thus reducing the cost in your telephone bill and online charges. The best you can get in a two-way modem using ordinary phone lines is 33,600 bits per second (bps). (A new technology called x2, lets you download information at 56,000 bps from specially equipped Internet service providers.)

> **TECHNO TALK**
>
> **Dot Matrix** is a fairly basic, but flexible printer. It can produce text or graphics in the form of a matrix of small dots, with each character formed by a series of pins striking a ribbon. They are generally used for jobs where the quality of the printing is not crucial.
>
> **Inkjet** printers can be described as the 'poor man's' laser printers (See above). The inkjet printing system prints characters and graphics by firing ink drops at the paper from thin nozzles. These printers use replaceable ink cartridges that contain both the print heads and the ink.
>
> **Laser** printers are fast, flexible and sophisticated devices that produce high quality printing. They work on similar principles to a photocopier, using a photo-sensitive drum, and can produce between 4 and 20 pages per minute.

Modems typically connect between your computer and your telephone line. However, if you have Cable Internet service available in your area, then you will find a cable modem a worthy alternative. These units plug into your cable television outlet and allow you to download data at up to 1.5 million bps – 25 times faster than the fastest telephone modems. However, there is a hefty monthly service charge attached to it.

Although you can get by with a 28,800 bps modem, you will find it slower. So, if you are buying a new phone modem and can afford it, go for a 33,600 bps modem with x2 capability. However, do make sure you check the connection speed offered by your service provider. If you decide to go for cable modem, get the one your cable TV company recommends.

WARNING!

Incoming calls and call waiting

```
. . . if someone picks up an extension phone while you are logged in, it
usually breaks your connection.

. . . if you have call waiting you should turn it off while your modem is on
the phone. For touch-tone phone type *70, (don't forget the comma) in front of
the number of your Internet service provider in your communication software.
If you have a pulse-dial phone type 1170, before the phone number.
```

2.3.3 which type of telephone line?

You can use your ordinary single telephone line to connect to the Internet, but it must have a plug-in socket. The socket must be located fairly close to your computer. Using an adapter, you should be able to plug-in the modem and a telephone in the same socket. If you want people to still be able to phone you when you are surfing the net, then you will be wise to have a second telephone line.

ISDN line – If you really need faster access to the Internet, you can get an ISDN line. This stands for Integrated Services Digital Network. It is a different type of link to your Internet service provider. It replaces your modem with a new device called a 'Terminal Adapter' and it can operate at four times the speed of a 33,600 bps modem. Right now it is very expensive and complicated. Cable modems may make it obsolete.

2.3.4 which communication software?

Communication *software (or comms program)* enables your computer to communicate and exchange information with other computers that are linked by *modems.* There are several types of comms software. For example, *Windows95* comes with Exchange and HyperTerminal while *Windows 3.1* comes with

Terminal. When you purchase your modem it usually comes with its own comms software. Also, major service providers like CompuServe, supply their own comms software.

If you bought your computer from a dealer stating that the system is 'Internet ready', then everything would have been done by the person who installed the software. However, if you have, or are planning, to install a modem on your own computer, then you will need to set up the software yourself or get someone else to do it for you.

2.3.5 which internet service provider?

Finally, you need to find a way to connect to a computer that is part of the Internet. The service provider is your gateway to the net.

So what is a service provider? Several hundred large companies in the UK maintain networks that are linked to the Internet via dedicated communication lines. Many of them are willing to let people like you and I use their dedicated communication lines to access the Internet, typically free of charge. The company you choose to log to the Internet is your service provider. Selecting which service provider is right for you may not be that easy, but is nevertheless a decision that you will have to make. Service providers can be divided into two: *online* services and *(Local) Internet service providers.*

▷ **Online services** – This type of service provider offers much more than basic Internet access and consequently charges more. Online services are like an exclusive club. Once you sign up you will have access to a range of members-only areas such as discussion forums, chat groups and file libraries as well as access to the Internet. You will also have user-friendly interface, special features unique to that provider, better security, longevity, and lots of user support. See Appendix 2 for a brief outline of the major players. Online services sound pretty good, but it could cost more than you are willing to pay. Read on, as there are other alternatives.

▷ **Local Internet service providers** (ISPs) – The two most popular kinds of accounts are Terminal or UNIX shell accounts and SLIP/PPP accounts.

With a terminal or UNIX shell account, your computer does not interact with Internet computers. You dial into your service provider's computer to indirectly connect to the Internet. Shell accounts are limited in features but less expensive than direct access accounts.

With SLIP or PPP account, you dial into a service provider's computer and run applications that directly connect you to the Internet. With this kind of direct connection your computer can use browsers with user-friendly graphical interfaces, such as NetScape, Internet Explorer or Eudora to interact with Internet computers. **SLIP** or **PPP** access to the Internet offers more performance and convenience than a shell account and cost a bit more.

SLIP (short for Serial Line Internet Protocol) and PPP (short for Point-to-Point Protocol), are Internet standards for transmitting Internet Protocol (IP) packets over serial lines (phone lines). Internet information is packaged into IP packets (a method for enclosing data into small, transmissible units wrapped up on one end, unbundled on the other). A service provider might offer SLIP, PPP, or both. Your computer must use connection software (usually provided by the service provider) that matches the protocol of the server's connection software. PPP is a more recent and robust protocol than SLIP. So if you have a choice, select PPP.

NOTE

Shell account vs SLIP or PPP account

Direct connection such as SLIP or PPP lets you download files directly to your system from remote sites. Whilst with indirect connection such as Shell account when you download a file from an Internet site, the file is saved on the service provider's computer. You then have to transfer the file from the service provider's computer to your home system.

Here are a few reasons to consider ISP:

- Lower cost; many providers offer a flat monthly rate (plus your telephone bill, of course);

- Choice of tools to access the Internet eg, NetScape, Eudora, and so on;

- Less censorship;

- You can normally choose the personalised part of your e-mail.

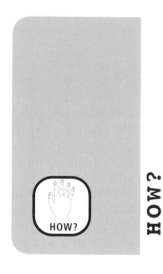

HOW?

How does an account with a service provider work?

The ISP provides you with a dial-up phone number. This phone number is called PoP (Point of Presence) (Fig 2.1). Using the software provided you dial-up the number to establish a link and the ISP routes you into the Internet.

Large Internet Service Providers have several PoPs. These are scattered across the country, thus providing users the facility of access using local calls, while others have only one PoP which may not be close to you.

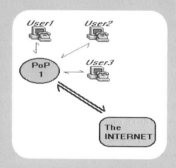

fig.2.1 **An illustration of a PoP**

2.3.6 taking out a subscription with which isp?

NOTE

Remember, there is no such thing as a perfect service provider – all of them are good for some people, bad for others. It is perfectly reasonable, therefore, to try several services before picking the one you like best. Also, Service Providers like the SUN, PC WORLD and a few others offer free access to the Internet.

There are loads of ISPs (Internet Service Providers) and a few online services in the UK. New ones are popping up all the time. Check the business pages in your local newspaper. For your convenience I have listed some of these providers in Appendix 2.

Choosing a provider can be a skill in itself. There are a few things to consider and a few questions to ask. Good service providers will be willing to provide you with straight answers. Here are eight points to guide you.

1 **Charges** – Check out for hidden charges. For example, if they charge extra for the time you spend online, make sure you do take this into consideration.

2 **Connection** – Seek past or present subscribers' opinion as to the reliability and availability of the system, especially during peak periods.

3 **Location of the PoP** – Enquire if the computer you are dialling into (the PoP) is local. Since the largest single cost you will face in using the Internet is your telephone bill, it's very important that you choose a provider who has a PoP as close to you as possible. If you are not able to dial-in using a local phone number, then forget it and try another provider.

④ **Modem speeds** – Check the speed of the modem the service provider is using. If you have a fast modem eg, 33.6Kbps, you do not want to connect to a service provider who uses a slower modem.

⑤ **PPP connection** – Enquire if you can choose PPP connection as opposed to SLIP connection. The former is faster and easier to set up.

⑥ **Software** – Many companies will send you preconfigured connection software that's ready to install. Ask about availability of technical telephone support if you get stuck.

⑦ **Subscription fees** – Find out the monthly subscription fee (if any), inclusive of VAT. If this ISP charges more, ask what else they provide that other companies don't. Enquire if you can pay annually, as this may be cheaper.

⑧ **Support** – Ensure that there is appropriate support for your system. (If you are an IBM user, you should expect your provider to offer wholehearted support for IBM Internet applications.) Also, check that good telephone support is available and whether there is a charge, particularly when you are most likely to need it, ie, during evenings and weekends.

2.3.7 signing up with an isp

On taking up a subscription with a provider, you will be given an account name. Providers differ in their approach to account names. Some just assign you a name, while others allow you some degree of choice, as long as the name has not already been used. It is important that you choose an account name that you like, because your account name will often form the unique part of your e-mail address, and this is the way you will be known to the rest of the world. Also you will need to quote your account name when you call the support line. So try not to ask for names, like "chubbychops". While this may seem funny at first thought, you may regret it later on when you're using e-mail to apply for a job.

There are two or three common approaches to choosing an address. It's worth following these, as they're accepted as "normal" on the Internet.

▷ 1st approach is your initial(s) followed by your surname. For example, mine is "*sschellen*"

▷ 2nd approach is your initials. Eg, "*ssc*". Had there already been an "ssc" on the system, a number can be added, eg "*ssc1*".

▷ 3rd approach is your main forename followed by the first letter(s) of your surname. Eg "*sydc*". If this already exists on the system, then it could be "*sydch*".

Most providers are reluctant to change people's e-mail addresses after the account has already been set up. So a few minutes of thought beforehand can avoid a lot of hassle later.

The rules on account names vary a little between providers. Usually they are lower-case, can't contain spaces, and often restricted to eight characters. Most importantly, another subscriber must not have already chosen it.

How does one get an account for a system at home?

For your home system, once you have chosen your Internet service provider, get on the phone and tell them you would like to subscribe. The provider will then set up an account for you. What happens next would vary from provider to provider.

▶ They may send you an account, followed by a disk preconfigured for your computer with instructions for installation.

▶ They may send you a disk of software, written instructions on how to install it and how to configure your computer, and some useful documentation.

If you have decided to subscribe with an online service provider, your first job is to get your hands on a free connection software. Phone them and request the correct software for your computer (see Appendix 2 for telephone numbers).

If a disk is supplied, somewhere on it you will be told how to start the program that signs you up, and the whole process will advance in simple steps.

Usually you will be able to try the service for 30 days. After you have keyed in all required details, the program will dial-up the service's computer and automatically set up your subscription. After a few minutes you should received a username and password.

How do I use an online service?

When you dial-in to your online service and log on using your username and password, you won't actually be on the Internet. You will find the main screen displaying a series of buttons. To access the Internet, you will need to click on a button clearly labelled Internet.

2.4 janet and the world wide web

As mentioned already JANET (Joint Academic Network) is the academic network of UK universities. It is designed for academic use by staff and students. As a healthcare student you are eligible to apply for a JNDS (JANET National Dial-up Service) account with **U-NET**. It is a service seriously worth considering. So, before you rush out to take a subscription with any ISPs or online services, you should enquire at the Computing services department of your college about a JNDS account. If you already have a JNDS account, you should be able to do at least five things. Activity 2.4 will help you to identify them.

Here are the five things you should be able to do with a JNDS account, for an annual flat rate fee, with no hourly charges or time limits. Use the checklist to tick (✓) those that you can do.

- ○ Pick up your college/university e-mail from home;
- ○ Access and surf the Net for all kinds of information;
- ○ 'Chat' directly to other Internet users;
- ○ Obtain high quality, high speed access to JANET to do your research or other projects from the comfort of your home;
- ○ Use 5Mb of webspace – for your hobbies, CV or other pleasures.

If you are able to do all the above and possibly more, you are doing well. Otherwise, you should have a serious chat with the Service Provider. You should also be provided with all the software you need to get online, calls are at local rate, technical support in the evenings and on Saturdays, and you should have a choice of e-mail addresses that you can take anywhere and keep after you leave education.

summary and conclusion

You will need an account to get online. Once you have obtained this, you must guard your password. If you are using your college/university NT workstation, this gives you free unlimited access to the Net, so use it as much as you can. If you are purchasing your own PC then go for the higher-end machine within your buying range, especially the modem. After you have chosen a good Internet Service Provider you are ready to surf away.

the world wide web

3

"Before I knew how to use the Internet, I was always behind with my projects because I just could not find the books I needed in the library. But, I can tell you this: the Net is so unbelievable. Now that I have access to so much information, I am never late with any of my assignments."

Student on Diploma of Education (Nursing Studies)
Canterbury Christ Church University College

"The World Wide Web is one of the most immediate and easy-to-use services on the Internet."

Hoyler (1996)[3]

URL (pronounced 'earl') is the unique 'address' of a file on the Internet.

A **browser** is a computer program that enables you to view web pages on the Internet. Although the NetScape browser is very popular, Microsoft Internet Explorer is catching up and is likely to become very popular, particularly with home users. The main advantage of Internet Explorer is that Microsoft gives it away for free, while NetScape Navigator/Communicator is a commercial software package. There are things that NetScape Navigator/Communicator can do and Internet Explorer can't, and vice versa, but in general they are equally powerful.

The World Wide Web ('web' or 'WWW', for short) is so easy to use that it has become the most popular service on the Internet. It is probably the reason for the 'Internet explosion'. To access the information on the web you need a piece of software. NetScape Navigator/Communicator is one of two major software programs that do the job well. The other major competitor is Internet Explorer. In this book, the screenshots have been taken from both Internet Explorer* and NetScape Navigator so that users of either program can compare the similarities. One of the big advantages of the web is that you do not need a menu. You use the hypermedia links embedded in web documents to thread your way through all types of related information. You can also access any document you want directly by entering its location through a **URL** (Uniform Resource Locator). In this unit we will identify some important features of a **browser** and how to use it to explore the web.

*The Internet Explorer program used for this book was provided by Freeserve, hence the FS logo on the top right-hand side of all screenshots.

checklist

Below is a checklist of what you can expect to find out in this Unit. Read through the statements then tick (✓) the items about which you would like to know more.

I would like to find out more about:

Please turn over the page and read through the topics you have ticked

Hypertext is a system of clickable texts used on the web. These clickable texts serve as a cross reference to another part of the document (or an entirely different document).

The web, developed by CERN (European Laboratory of Particle Physics) in Switzerland, is a system that uses the Net to link together vast quantities of information all over the world. It is made up of a series of "*pages*", containing both text and graphics. Some of the words or phrases are underlined and highlighted in a different colour from the text around them. These are called **hypertext** or hyperlinks. If you place your mouse-pointer on to one of these hyperlinks (you'll see it change into a hand with a pointing finger) and click the mouse button, you will be transported to either a new section of the text or a brand-new document.

NOTE

A web page is a single document that can be any length, like a document in a word processor. Pages can contain text, graphics, sound and video-clips, together with clever effects and controls.

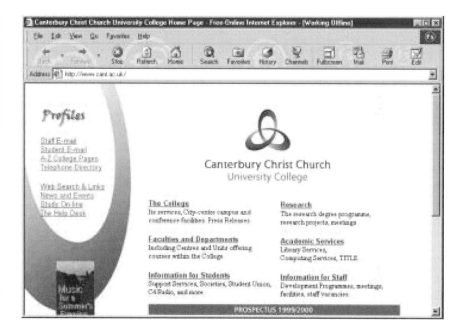

▷ fig. 3.1 **A web page showing hyperlinks**

By moving your mouse-pointer over coloured hypertext and clicking your mouse-button, you can jump between pages of related documents.

3.1.1 the nature of hypertext and hyperlinks

NOTE

The 'web' is developing all the time, and is likely to become the biggest library on earth – an invaluable resource for any health student doing research or completing course assignments.

Here are a few points to remember about these two features of web pages:

▷ These hyperlinks are not restricted to opening documents stored on the same computer. You could be reading a page stored on a computer in Kent, and clicking a hypertext could take you to a page stored on another computer in Australia.

▷ Hypertext links are not always a word or phrase. Sometimes there is a picture that you click on, or a part of a larger picture, with different parts linking to different pages.

▷ Besides opening a new web page, a link sometimes would display a picture, download a program, play a video or a sound, run a program and so on . . .

HOW?

3.1.2 storage of web pages

The web is made up of many millions of files placed on computers called web
servers. Although no one person or company owns the web itself, the web servers
are owned by different companies. They either rent or give away free space to
anyone who wants to put their own pages on the web. These pages are created
using a text-based language called HTML (HyperText Markup Language). Once
these newly created pages are available on the web, anyone who knows their
address can read them.

Simple web pages can be created in minutes. Thus, a **web site** can be as up-
to-date as its creator wants it to be. Some are updated more frequently than others.

Web site is a
term loosely used
to refer to *web
pages* belonging to
an individual or organisation.
A site could be a single page or
several complex pages belonging
to a University, College, Hospital
Trust or a Nurse Therapist.

3.1.3 web browsers

As already mentioned, to view pages on the WWW and information from
other Internet resources, you'll need to use a *browser*. The browser that you use
determines how the web information is displayed. Some browsers provide a text-
only feature and cannot display the richer content of web files that may include
graphics, video or audio clips. There are a number of these available. No matter
which browser you use, you will be able to access thousands of research sources
to complete your health projects. The only things you might miss are the effects
of multimedia presentation. In this book we will concentrate on Microsoft
Internet Explorer for two reasons: firstly it is a browser which is becoming very
popular, especially with home users, and secondly, it is the one that has recently been adopted at Canterbury Christ Church University College and is likely to
become the standard in other colleges.

When the browser is activated the first page is loaded and displayed on the
screen. This starter-screen is known as the 'homepage'. A homepage – like the
one shown in Fig. 3.2 – serves two purposes: it allows the college to present an
image of what the institution is about, and it lets you and other students and staff
establish links to other sites of interest. For example, in Canterbury Christ Church
University College (CCCUC) homepage you will find hyperlinks to various pages
created by the college, and to other web sites around the world. If you are not at
CCCUC, the homepage at your institution will look different and will provide a
completely different set of links since each site's homepage defines the links it
feels are most appropriate.

NOTE

. . . students from other
institutions can visit CCCUC by
entering this website address in
the Address/Location box:
http://www.cant.ac.uk

3.1.4 starting your browser

Address or Location box It is the box where you type your favourite web site addresses. In Internet Explorer this box is labelled 'Address' while in NetScape Navigator it is labelled 'Location'

Before you can start using some of the features on your browser you must first be connected to the Net. This is fairly easy to do in a Windows environment if you are able to use a mouse. It is just a matter of identifying the appropriate icon and double-clicking on it with your mouse. If you are not sure how to gain access to the Net, the next activity will help you do so. When you reach the homepage, take a good look at your browser and make a special mental note of the **Address** or **Location** box.

activity 3.1   LOGGING ON AND OFF THE INTERNET ON THE COLLEGE NETWORK

I am assuming in this book that you have the program 'Microsoft Internet Explorer or NetScape Navigator/Communicator' installed on your WINDOWS NT WORKSTATION. If this is the case, follow the step-by-step instructions listed in **Worksheet 1**, they will help you get ON and OFF the Internet. Please complete both the logging ON and OFF.

If you're using NetScape Navigator/Communicator or something else, you should find that most of the facilities available on Microsoft Internet Explorer are also available in other browsers, and many of them can be accessed by similar toolbar buttons, menu options or keystrokes.

When you have completed the activity return to this page and read on

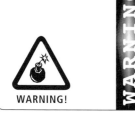

WARNING!

If you are unable to identify the Microsoft Internet Explorer icon to start the program (or the icon of the browser installed on the system you are using), you should seek help immediately. You should find the Help desk in your institution quite accommodating.

Starting your browser

NetScape
Navigator

Internet
Explorer

① Log on to Windows NT now (if you have not already done so).

② Identify the **NetScape or Internet Explorer** icon.

③ Using the mouse, **double-click** on the icon. *This should start the browser program and – if all goes well – the homepage of **your** service provider (or your institution) should be loaded and displayed on the screen.*

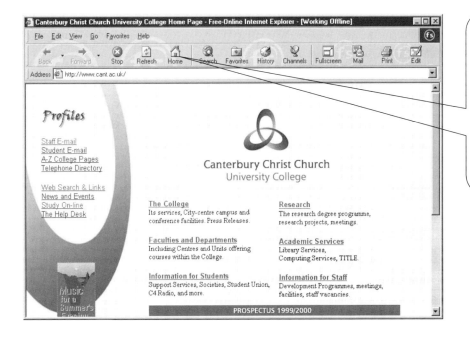

fig. 3.2 **The homepage of Canterbury Christ Church University College**

> **Comment**
>
> Don't worry if what you see on your screen looks slightly different to the screenshot on the left.
>
> The homepage is where you will start exploring the web. You can return to the homepage at anytime by clicking on the 'Home' button on the tool bar.

Quitting the Internet

① Point and click on the command **File**. *A submenu should appear.*

② Point and click on the command **Close/Exit**. *You should be back to Windows Program Manager or Windows Desktop.*

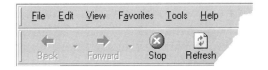

> **Comment**
>
> You have just arrived online, and you are eager to explore. There are a few things more I need to tell you before you start your adventure. So let's get off the Net for now and continue reading Unit 3. To quit follow the steps on the left.

NOTE

Although there are a number of browsers (some available in several versions), most share some common features.

Having carried out Activity 3.1 above, you would have noticed the 'Homepage' displayed by your browser. It may have resembled in some way the homepage in the screenshot below. You may also have noticed some of the features of your browser and of the web page. These may not have made much impression on you. However, they are features that you will be using over and over when exploring the web and surfing the Net. So let's get acquainted with the basic workings of a browser and the web itself.

Buttons on the toolbar allow you to navigate between pages, point you to interesting places and enable you to refresh a web page's content. Most of the buttons on the Internet Explorer also appear on NetScape Navigator.

This white box shows the address of the current page. It is also the box where you can type your favourite Web addresses (URLs). In *Internet Explorer* this box is labelled 'Address' whilst in *NetScape Navigator* it is labelled 'Location'.

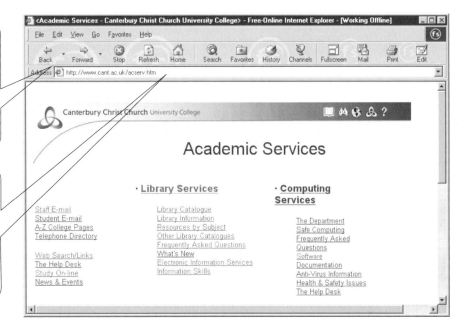

fig. 3.3 **some important features of a browser**

3.1.5 anatomy of a web page

If you look at the homepage shown above you should be able to see several *hypertext links* (ie, underlined, coloured text). When you move your screen-pointer on to any link and click on it, your browser sends a message to the server storing the page that you have requested. Then, if everything goes according to plan, the server responds by sending back the requested page so that your browser can display it. Links that you have visited before are (usually) in red; those which you have not visited are (usually) in blue. Figure 3.4 shows another screenshot. We can use this as an example to highlight the type of thing you will find on a web page, which are as follows:

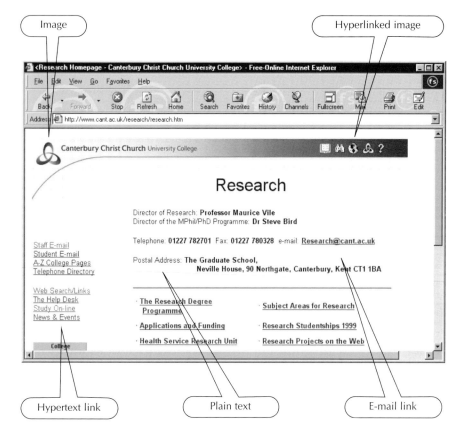

◁ fig. 3.4 **some elements that make up a web page**

▶ **Plain text** – This is ordinary readable text. Clicking on it will have no effect.

▶ **Plain Image** – A picture or graphic that simply enhances a web site and it won't lead anywhere if you click on it.

▶ **Hypertext links** – Text links to other places ("hotlinks"). Text links are nearly always underlined and their text colour is usually red, after they have been visited. Clicking on these will route you to a related topic.

▶ **Hyperlink images** – These do the same thing as hypertext link. In most cases they look no different to ordinary images, but they may be outlined in red or blue or the same colour as any hypertext links on the page.

▶ **E-mail link** – Click on this link and you will be able to send an e-mail message to the web page's author. The author's address will be automatically inserted into the message for you.

3.1.6 world wide web addresses (urls)

Every page on the web has its own individual address (URL), which tells your web browser where to find it. The standard format used for specifying the desired URL is composed of four simple components that identify the critical elements needed to access a document. Below is the URL of a government department: it is the homepage of the English Department of Health. Incidentally, it has details of, amongst other things, the Health of the Nation plus updates and research findings. Let's use the URL http://www.open.gov.uk/doh/dhome.htm to examine the four components.

TRANSFER FORMAT	HOST COMPUTER	DIRECTORY PATH	FILENAME
http://	www.open.gov.uk/	Doh/	dhhome.htm
1	2	3	4

Hosts *are* computers that are directly connected to the Internet.

▷ In Table 3.1, the first part of the URL is the transfer format. It indicates a hypertext (ie, a web page) and tells your browser the transfer format that will be needed. (Table 3.2 shows some common transfer formats.)

▷ The second part of the URL is the name of the **host** computer on which the web page is stored. Note that it is separated from the transfer format by a colon(:) and two forward slashes (//).

▷ The third part of the URL is the directory path on the host computer where the web page is stored. Note that the components of the directory location are separated from each other with a single forward slash (/), not the backslash (\) that some other operating systems expect.

▷ The fourth and final part of the URL is the name of the file containing a hypertext document. In our example it is the homepage of the Department of Health in the United Kingdom. Web documents are usually given the extension **.html** or **.htm**.

WARNING!

It is important that when typing a URL you match capitalisation and spelling in any component correctly. The slightest typing error will prevent your browser from fetching the document you requested.

3.1.7 some common service types

Most URLs start with "http://", which means that they are ordinary WWW addresses (the "http" stands for "Hypertext Transfer Protocol", which is the system NetScape uses to fetch WWW pages). There is an older and simpler service that you may find, called "*Gopher*" (For additional information read Section 7.3). You may encounter Gopher sites if you look at University information systems; Internet Explorer and NetScape are quite happy to handle them. The URL of a Gopher site will begin with "gopher://". It's also possible to use your web browser to access anonymous FTP sites (see Section 7.1), in which case the URL will begin with "ftp://". There are a couple of other service types – especially Usenet news ("news:"), or e-mail ("mailto:") (for additional information read Unit 6).

TRANSFER FORMAT SPECIFICATION	SERVER ACCESSED
http://	World Wide Web
https://	WWW with secure links
gopher://	Gopher
ftp://	FTP
news:	USENET
mailto:	e-mail

◁ table 3.2 **Common transfer formats**

The following is a short list of other mysterious things you will see in URLs:

- **.html** or **.htm** is the filename extension for a hypertext document.
- **Index.html** is the master page of a web site.
- **.Txt** is a plain text document without links.
- **.Gif** or **.jpg** or **.jpeg** is a picture
- **www** is short for World Wide Web

3.1.8 domain names

Every site on the Internet, whether accessed by WWW, e-mail, FTP etc., is addressed by the Internet "domain name".

A domain name is composed a bit like an address on an envelope. It is composed of several parts strung together with periods. Domain names are usually decoded from left to right. In the URL we looked at above, the domain name is:

http://www.open.gov.uk

The **.uk** shows that the site is in the UK. A site in Denmark ends with **.dk**; a site in China ends with **.cn**. An Australian site uses **.au** or sometimes, for historical reasons **.oz**; a site in India ends with **.in**. Some domain names don't end with a country code: these are usually (but not always) in the USA. There is a **.us** domain, but it's not often used – the Americans don't put their country on their domains for a similar reason to why we in the UK don't put the country on our stamps – they were there first. Also United Kingdom uses uk instead of the country code GB. Appendix 3 offers a comprehensive list of countries that have Internet connection and their country code.

The next domain, in our example above, to the left is **.gov**, which indicates a government institution (sometimes they use **.govt**). A commercial organisation uses **.co**, a similar US site would use **.com**. An academic organisation such as a university would use **.ac** (or in the US, **.edu**). A school uses **.sch**, a non-profit organisation uses **.org**, and backbone Internet organisations use **.net**.

Anything to the left of the organisation name is up to the organisation to assign – in the example above, the **www.open** identifies the particular computer within the organisation which handles the World Wide Web.

NOTE

Host and domain names are important because they can help you to infer something more about new resources as they are discovered. For example information from a UK organisation ought to have more authority than one located on a US organisation computer.

NOTE

A link you've visited before will be displayed in a different colour (usually red rather than blue). Also, most Web pages will have more information in them than can be seen comfortably on a screen. Use the 'scroll bars' at the right and underneath the page to move up-and-down and left-and-right within a page.

When you view a web page using your browser, you will see that it contains information and "hotlinks". These are underlined, like this:

▷ To follow the hotlink (ie, a key phrase or word) you simply place your mouse-pointer on it and click the mouse-button.

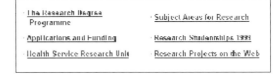

◁ With these buttons you can retrace your steps. For example, you can click on the '**Back**' button to go back a page or more. When you have gone back, you can click on the '**Forward**' button to go to the next page again. To return to the Homepage, simply click on the '**Home**' button.

▷ Your browser keeps track of the pages you have visited in your current session. At any time you can go back to an earlier page by using the "**Go**" command located on the menu bar.

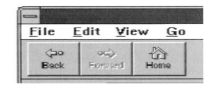

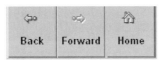

◁ While pages are being fetched you will be entertained by a lightning storm around the 'Internet Explorer' or 'NetScape' icon. Fetching pages can take quite a long time – especially from overseas. At busy periods the Internet can get swamped, and at these times you may lose patience with the slow speed at which, for example, pictures can be retrieved. Just point and click on the '**Stop**' button to interrupt your browser.

3.2.1 internet explorer toolbar

In Activity 3.2 below you will be navigating the web. You will no doubt notice a few more features on your browser's toolbar and wonder about their functions. So, here is a quick review:

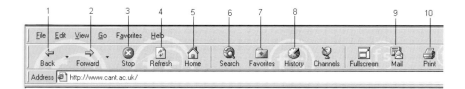

fig. 3.5 **The Internet Explorer toolbar and address box for typing URLs**

1 **Back** Clicking this button will take you back to the last page you looked at. If you keep clicking you can step all the way back to the first page.

2 **Forward** After going back, you can go forward again (to the next page you looked at) with this forward button. This button will be greyed-out if you haven't used the Back button yet.

3 **Stop** At busy periods it could take a long time before a page is loaded. If you have lost patience, click on the 'Stop' button to interrupt Internet Explorer or NetScape Navigator.

4 **Refresh** Sometimes things go wrong. Click this button and your browser will start downloading the same page again. (On NetScape Navigator this button is labelled **Reload**.)

5 **Home** As explained already, the homepage is where you will start exploring the web. You can return to the homepage at any time by clicking on the 'Home' icon.

6 **Search** Clicking on this button will let you specify a word or phrase to locate within the current Internet Explorer page. You can specify case sensitivity and search direction. If a match is found, the text is selected and displayed. (On NetScape Navigator this button is labelled **Find**.)

7 **Favorites** See *Bookmarks* 3.2.3 below.

8 **History** Click on this icon and you will see a list of all the sites you have visited. In most cases you should be able to revisit these sites offline.

8 **Mail** This opens a menu from which you can run your e-mail or news-reader software, or open a blank form to send an e-mail message.

10 **Print** Prints the current page. A dialogue box lets you select printing characteristics.

NOTE

Apart from numbers 7, 8 and 9 all the features described on the Internet Explorer toolbar also appear on the rival browser – NetScape Navigator toolbar – and they perform the same functions.

EXPLORING THE WEB activity **3.2**

Now that you know a few things about your browser, let's start using it to make an initial exploration of the Web.

▷ The step-by-step instructions listed in **Worksheet 2** should help you to follow a few links and to skip from page to page casually. If you find yourself going down a blind alley, use the tools '*Home*', '*Back*', '*Forward*' and '*Stop*' discussed above to retrace your steps, and move in a different direction.

▷ If you are an absolute beginner to the Internet, don't try to overdo it on this initial visit. Contain yourself to using the tools discussed so far.

When you have completed the activity return to the next page and read on

worksheet **2**   exploring the world wide web

NetScape Navigator

Internet Explorer

Charting your course

1. Log on to Windows NT as you did before.

2. Identify the **Internet Explorer** or **NetScape** icon.

3. Using the mouse, **double-click** on the icon. *This should start the browser program and – if all goes well – the homepage of **your** service provider (or your institution) should be loaded and displayed on the screen.*

4. Point and click on any hotlink you want to explore.

5. Now, follow the hotlink and other hotlinks until you are ready to stop. Practice using the following buttons on your toolbar: **BACK**, **FORWARD**, **STOP** and **HOME**.

6. When you are ready to finish, close down your browser, then log off Windows.

3.2.2 address or location box

'*URL*' is just a convoluted term for 'address'. You might have already noticed that the URL of the current page is shown in the 'Address' or 'Location' box. Every time you open a new page, its URL appears in the Address/Location box.

If you know the location (ie, the URL) of a page, you can go directly to it. You simply type it into the location box and press the ENTER key (on your keyboard). For example, if you are interested in oncology and need information on cancer you can go directly to the Cancer Oncolink site by typing this URL:

http://cancer.med.upenn.edu

At this site you will find information on many different types of cancer and the latest treatment, and much more.

In the next Activity I will give you a few URLs to enter and you will be able to follow up some useful sites.

3.2.3 hotlists

As you work with the Internet sites, you are going to discover places that you will want to revisit frequently. Rather than typing the address each time you need to access the site, you can add it to a list and your browser will remember this list between sessions. Internet Explorer refers to this hotlist as **Favorites** while NetScape Navigator calls it **Bookmarks**. The steps for creating a hotlist are quite easy. The next activity will show you how to do this. But first, here is the process (Fig. 3.6).

fig. 3.6 **How to create a hotlist**

Creating a hotlist in Internet Explorer

▷ Select "Add to Favorites" from the Favorites menu to add the current page to your Favorites list.

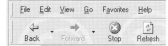

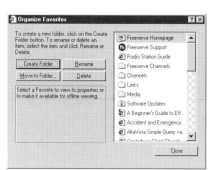

◁ Internet Explorer allows you to organise your shortcuts into submenus to make them easy to find. You simply select the file or files, then click one of the buttons to organise them.

Creating a hotlist in NetScape Navigator

▷ Select "Add Bookmark" from the Bookmark menu to add the current page to your bookmark list

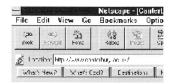

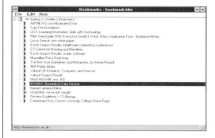

◁ NetScape's "Bookmarks" window allows you to drag elements in your bookmark list around, and insert headers and separators.

▷ If you select an element in the Bookmark window and choose "Properties" from the "Item" menu, you get this window which allows you to rename the bookmark and add notes.

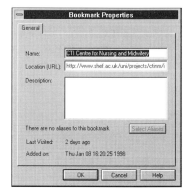

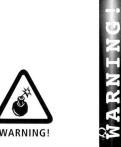

When you are trying to open a web page you may experience problems. For example, at the time you requested a page, the server may not be running or it may be busy. In both cases your browser may respond with a message 'time out', and in the latter case you may get a part of the page and then everything seems to have stopped. In the case of the latter, you may be able to get things moving by clicking the reload (refresh) button on your browser's toolbar. This will get your browser to try again. This may be sufficient to solve the problem, but be prepared to give up and try again later.

There is also the problem of the 'Vanishing Page Syndrome'. Although all web pages contain links, sometimes the pages those links refer to no longer exist and you will receive an error message instead. This is because the web is constantly changing, hence pages (or even sites) move elsewhere, are renamed, or simply disappear.

So, some of the URLs included in this book may have expired by the time you get to try them. This is, unfortunately, part of the magic of the web.

3.2.4 exchanging hotlists

Both Internet Explorer (IE) and NetScape Navigator keep your hotlist in a folder/file on the hard disk. The folder in IE is called "**Favorites**" and is stored in Windows directory; while in NetScape Navigator the file is called "**BOOK-MARK.HTM**". Both files can be read by other web browsers.

If you want to send your hotlist to a friend, this is not as difficult as you may think. Simply locate and copy the file on to a floppy disk or if you want it to go by e-mail, enclose it as an attachment (See the section on e-mail).

Both browsers have the ability to import any **.htm** file, extract the hotlinks, and put them in your Favorite/Bookmark list. Thus if while surfing the web you find a list of links which interest you, just save the page as a .htm file by using the "**Save As . . .**" option from your browser.

Now that we have covered a bit more about the WWW, you should have sufficient understanding of it, and how to navigate your way around with a reasonable degree of confidence and satisfaction. So let's try another activity.

activity 3.3 ENTERING URLS AND ADDING INTERESTING SITES TO YOUR HOTLIST

> ▶ Read **Section 3.3**, taking special notice of the caution given in the warning box.
> ▶ Select a few sites you would like to visit.
> ▶ Use the step-by-step instructions in **Worksheet 3** and start trying out all or at least some of the web addresses you have selected from the list offered.
> ▶ Add those sites you want to revisit later on to a hotlist (For help refer to **Worksheet 4**).

3.3 selected uk and foreign web sites applicable for nursing and allied professions

More and more sites of interest are emerging all the time. Once you become familiar with the Net you will no doubt discover all the sites you care to discover. You will find bloated volumes of directories of web sites in your library or bookshop. You will also find some web pages listing interesting web sites. I have gathered a list of useful UK and foreign sites and organised them under the following thirteen headings that you should find helpful when searching for information for your coursework.

> ▶ Organisations, associations and UK statutory bodies
> ▶ Adult nursing and medicine

- Alternative medicine
- General health information
- Mental health nursing, psychiatry and learning disabilities
- Midwifery and health visiting
- Paediatric nursing and medicine
- Paramedical
- Healthcare research
- Journals for health professions
- Libraries and free health databases
- Electronic publication and citation
- Quality of public services

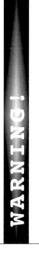

WARNING!

Each of the sites listed in this book have been checked on several occasions to ensure there have been no changes to site addresses since this book was first submitted for publication. As the web is still growing, it is possible that some sites might restructure their information as they add new areas of content. If you should find an address to which you could not connect, you should try connecting to the host system without specifying a specific document for viewing. In other words, if the site in the book is listed like this:

<u>http://www.scilib.uci.edu/~martindale/HSGuide.html</u>

you might try connecting to this address:

<u>http://www.scilib.uci.edu</u>

You can then look through the main content areas at the site to see if you can find the information in a new location.

ENTERING URLS   worksheet **3**

The Internet is growing all the time. Hoyler (1997) reports that over 100 new WWW sites are added each day. In Section 3.3, I have listed a series of URLs of Internet sites for nursing and the allied professions which you can visit and evaluate their usefulness for yourself. All you will need to do is to type any chosen URL into your web browser's Address/Location box and press the ENTER key on your keyboard. See steps below.

ENTERING URLS

① Log on to Windows NT and then start your Browser. *After a few seconds the homepage should appear.*

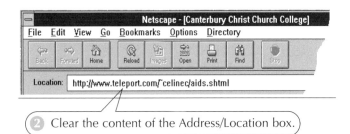

② Clear the content of the Address/Location box.

Comment

One way of clearing the content of the Address/Location box is to:

Place your mouse-pointer in the box and double-click on the (left) mouse button. *This should highlight the content of the box .*

Then press the BACKSPACE key on your keyboard. *The content of the box should vanish.*

③ (Select a URL from Section 3.3) or if you have one of your own, type it as shown in the screenshot on p. 42.

④ Make sure there are no typing errors, then press the **ENTER** key (on your keyboard). *If all goes well, after a while the requested page should load.*

WARNING!

Remember that fetching pages can take a long time — especially from overseas, and also at busy periods. So, be patient. If you are tired of waiting point and click on *'Stop'* button on the toolbar. Then try another address.

⑤ If you are absolutely sure you have typed the address correctly and have still received an error message, click on the '**Home**' button on the tool-bar and try another address.

worksheet 4

ADDING A WEB SITE ADDRESS TO A HOTLIST

For Internet Explorer
ADDING FAVORITE

① Point and click on the command **Favorites** on the menubar. *A submenu should appear.*

② Click on the command **Add to Favorites**. *An Add Favorite dialog box should appear.*

③ Click on the **OK** button. *The Add Favorite dialog box should disappear, and the URL of your current web page would have been added to your Favorites list.*

HOW?

To check that the URL of your current web page has indeed been added to your Favorites list, first click on the 'Home' button. Then click on the command 'Favorites' on the toolbar, and you should find a reference to the page you have stored. To load that page again, simply point and click on it.

For NetScape Navigator
ADDING BOOKMARK

① Point and click on the command **Bookmark** on the menubar. *A sub-menu should appear.*

② Click on the command **Add Bookmark**. *The submenu should close, and the URL of your current web page would have been added to your bookmark list.*

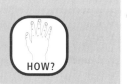

HOW?

To check that the URL of your current web page has indeed been added to your bookmark list, first click on the 'Home' button. Then repeat Step 1 above, and you should find a reference to the page you have stored. To load that page again, simply point and click on it.

associations, organisations, and UK statutory bodies

English National Board for Nursing, Midwifery and Health Visiting
http://www.enb.org.uk

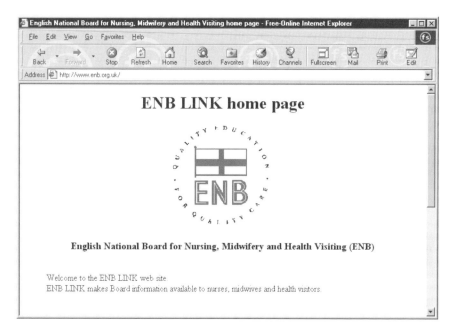

◁ At this site you will find all Board circulars, Board's Health Care Database, Regulations and Guidelines, pre- and post-registration careers information, a full text of free publications and lists of Board publications and how they can be purchased, information on Board-commissioned research, and information about specific practice areas, such as mental health nursing

AIDS /HIV: Terence Higgins Trust
http://www.tht.org.uk

This is the UK's leading HIV and AIDS charity web site. Here you will find an abundance of information in the world of HIV and AIDS. There is also a facility to request additional information.

Alzheimer's Association
http://www.alzheimers.org.uk

This site contains links to other resources and information on chapter contacts, conferences and events, and medicine and caregivers.

Anthony Nolan Trust
http://wombat.doc.ic.ac.uk/bone-marrow/index.html

This is a bone-marrow trust registered in the UK. It is a charity that exists to match volunteer bone marrow donors with patients throughout the world, who are in need of life-saving bone marrow transplants. At this site you will find information on bone-marrow, how to become a donor and much more.

Arthritis and Rheumatism Council

http://rheuma.bham.ac.uk/arc.html

This is a major UK charity dedicated to supporting research and education relating to joint diseases. The website has a range of information for patients, healthcare professionals and researchers.

CANCERHELP

http://medweb.bham.ac.uk/cancerhelp/public.bacup

This is a free service about cancer and cancer care for the general public and health professionals. The site contains information for kids, adults and health professionals.

British Computer Society Nursing Specialist Group

http://www.man.ac.uk/bcsnsg/index.html

This nursing specialist group is one of five Health Informatics Specialist Groups of the British Computer Society and contributes to the national and international debates on information management and technology issues within healthcare. At this site you will find information on all the focus groups.

British Digestive Foundation

http://www.bdf.org.uk/

This is the only national charity that is concerned with all forms of digestive disorders. The site provides information for sufferers, their families and friends.

Information for Health

http://www.imt4nhs.exec.nhs.uk/index.htm

▷ At this site you will find information strategy for the modern NHS. Information is organised under the following sections:

▶ Health service circular;
▶ Full strategy document;
▶ Executive summary;
▶ Short version information for health – New strategy presentation with speaker notes.

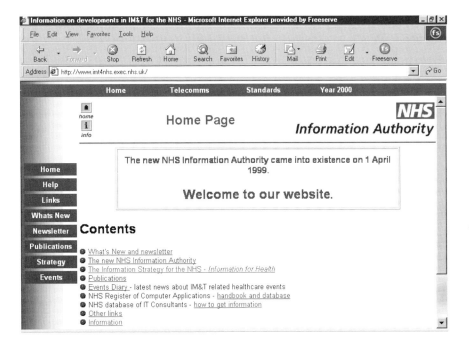

Deaf and Hard of Hearing

http://web.ukonline.co.uk/hearing.concern/

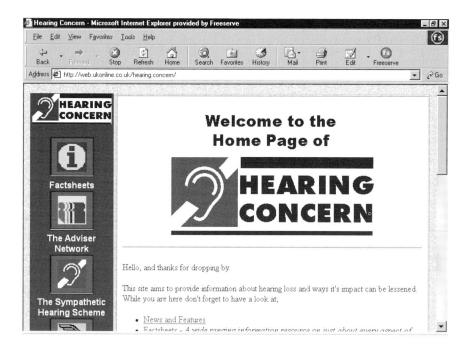

◁ This site provides information about hearing loss and ways its impact can be lessened. There is also a factsheet and other useful subsections.

Department of Health

http://www.open.gov.uk/doh/dhhome.htm

Homepage of the government department. Has details of, among other things, the Health of the Nation plus updates and research findings.

Diabetes: Adults

http://www.diabetic.org.uk/index.htm

This site brings together in one place information for people with diabetes.

Epilepsy

http://www.epilepsy.org.uk/

Here you will find all sorts of information on epilepsy. Information is organised under the following sections: Epilepsy a parents' guide; employment; self-management; women; medical management; leisure; education; driving.

Hepatitis Network

http://www.hepnet.com/

This is an excellent site. It has an interactive learning section that is quite easy to use. It will update you on almost everything you need to know about hepatitis. It also has a 'Quick Search' option.

Institute of Psychiatry

http://www.iop.kcl.ac.uk/

This site, amongst other things, has a useful 'Student Forum' section. A click on this section will link you to BIDS, BioMedNet, a selection of online journals and more.

Marie Stopes Institute
http://www.mariestopes.org.uk/

This site provides all sorts of information relating to people's right to have children by choice.

Mental Health Foundation
http://www.mentalhealth.org.uk/

This is the UK charity improving the lives of everyone with mental health problems or learning disabilities. At this site you will find links to various related sites.

Royal College of Nursing (RCN)
http://www.thebiz.co.uk

Human resources, training and development, membership and other information.

United Kingdom Central Council for Nurses
http://www.ukcc.org.uk

The regulatory body for the nursing, midwifery and health visiting professions throughout the UK.

Information for Dentalphobics
http://www.dentalfear.org/

▷ This page is written and published by Dr Stuart M. Ellis, Dental Surgeon, Cambridge, England. There is a lot of information on dental phobia and how to deal with it.

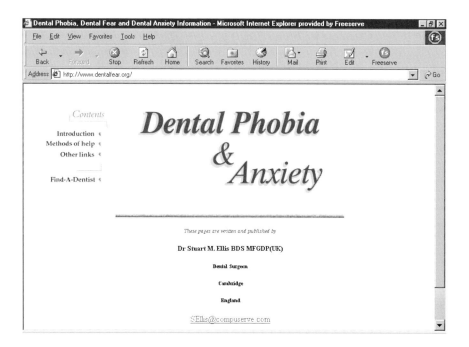

World Health Organization

http://www.who.ch/

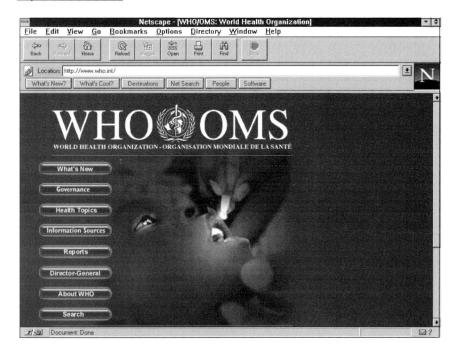

◁ Here you will find information about its own research, details about conferences, epidemiological reports and much more.

Multiple Sclerosis Society

http://www.mssociety.prg.uk/

This society supports people whose lives are affected by multiple sclerosis by funding research and provides local and national services. At this site you will find information on drug therapies, welfare publications and information for professionals. There is also a FAQ (Frequently Asked Questions) section.

National Board of Nursing, Midwifery and HV in Scotland

http://www.nbs.org.uk

This site is similar to its sister site – the English National Board. It contains various regulations and guidelines, the board publications and so on.

Prostate Help Association

http://www.u-net.com/~pha/

This is a registered charity. The site offers information on all types of prostate disease.

Spina Bifida and Hydrocephalus

http://www.asbah.demon.co.uk/ifhsb.html

Here you will find comprehensive information on Spina Bifida. There are also links to other related sites.

Twins and Multiple Births Association

http://www.surreyweb.org.uk/tamba/

This is a registered charity in the UK for all parents with twins, triplets, quads, quins, sextuplets or more. The site provides information and mutual support networks for families of twins or more.

Women's Health: Infertility
http://www.ferti.net/uk/index.htm

▷ This is a national awareness campaign site. It provides information on how to campaign and influence your MP, get more media coverage and set up a patient group. There are links to other sites.

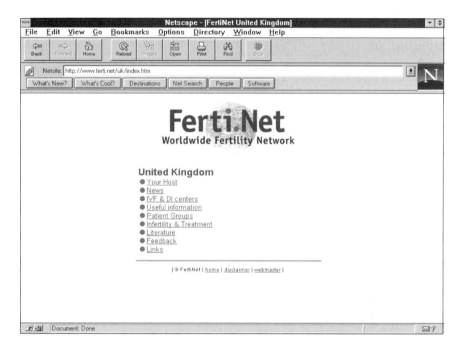

adult nursing and medicine

AIDS Information Service
http://oneworld.org/avert/

▷ This site offers information on preventative health education.

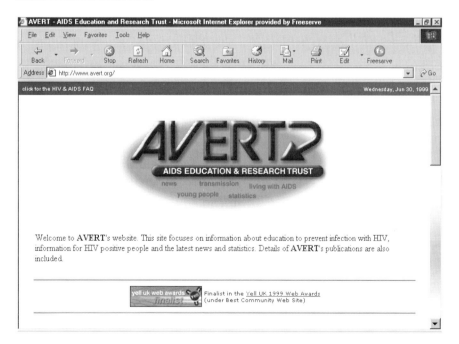

Ask Noah about Heart Disease

http://www.noah.cuny.edu/heart_disease/heartdisease.html

Here you will find answers to many questions about heart disease. The site includes Stroke Guide and information on anatomy, causes, types, statistics, and symptoms. There are also links to information on prevention, care and treatment, and resources.

AIDS Resource List

http://www.teleport.com/~celinec/aids.shtml

This is an extensive resource containing links to: AIDS glossary, AIDS Memorial Quilt website, AIDS Project for Teens, HIV Info web, AIDS in specific countries such as Mexico and France, AIDS prevention.

Alzheimer's Disease Resource Page

http://www.cwru.edu/orgs/adsc/intro.html

This site contains information for caregivers, physicians and researchers. General information resources include: common questions, a fact sheet, statistics, warning signs and ways to help Alzheimer's patients and their families.

Alzheimer's Web

http://werple.mira.net.au/~dhs/ad.html

This site provides patients and their families with the latest information available including answers to frequently asked questions about the disease and its biochemical pathology. You will also find information on the following: links to research laboratories and other homepages, books, articles, references and conferences.

Breast Cancer Information Clearing House

http://nysernet.org/bcic

At this site you will find information on: breast cancer detection, support groups, questions and answers, and other medical links.

Cancer Guide by a Recovered Cancer Patient

http://cancerguide.org

This is a guide put together by Steve Dunn who survived a diagnosis of cancer. He hopes his guide will help others.

Cancer OncoLink

http://cancer.med.upenn.edu

This site provides information on the many different types of cancer and the latest treatments. Topics include: psychosocial support, cancer causes and screening, clinical trials, frequently asked questions on cancer and financial issues for cancer patients.

CancerWeb

http://www.graylab.ac.uk/cancerweb.html

This site offers information on cancer.

Centres for Disease Control and Prevention

http://www.cdc.gov

At this site you can read about prevention strategies for various diseases. You can even get more into the details with the scientific data, surveillance information, and health statistics.

Explore the Virtual Heart

http://sln.fi.edu/biosci/heart.html

▷ At this site you will learn how:

❯ a drug-free lifestyle helps your heart,
❯ exercise helps your heart,
❯ healthy eating helps your heart,
❯ you and your doctor can monitor your heart.

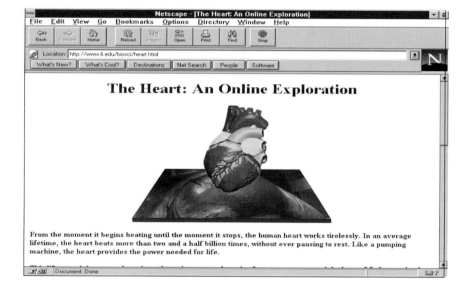

The Virtual Medical Centre

http://sun2.lib.uci.edu/HSG/Medical.html

▷ This site is primarily aimed at medical students. Nursing and allied students would also find it beneficial. It has pages with detailed information in many different areas such as:

❯ Endocrinology,
❯ Haematology,
❯ Ophthalmology,
❯ Orthopaedics,
❯ Urology and
❯ Virology

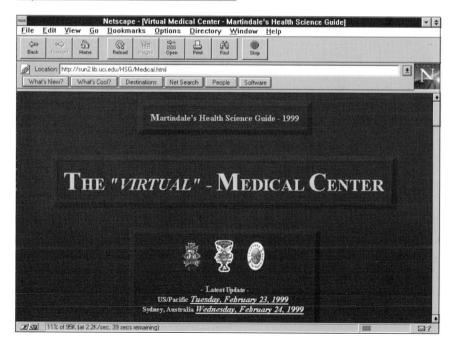

Cool Medical Site of the Week

http://www.graphics.stanford.edu/~lorensen/vw/vw.html

This includes marching through the visible woman, Jane's brain, and talking skeleton (click the bones and they speak).

Diabetes

http://www.adatx.org/diabetes.html

At this site you will find information from the American Diabetes Association.

First Aid Sites

http://www.healing-aid.com/links.html

You can consult this site for healthcare advice on emergency situations. Links include: emergency medicine and primary care homepage, what to do during life-threatening emergencies, injury control resource information network, and National Collegiate EMS Foundation Home Page.

Index – Infectious Disease

http://www.cc.emory.edu/WHSCL/medweb.id.html

At this site you can consult a variety of medical resources such as: Pathology and Virology Centre, Virtual Library of Diseases, World Wide Web Communicable Disease Resources. There is also a long list of sites for specific diseases.

Interactive Patient Home Page

http://medicus.marshall.edu/medicus.htm

Test your diagnostic skills.

International Cancer Information Centre

http://www.icic.nci.nih.gov

From this site you can access CancerNet for the latest information on cancer. You can also read news and abstracts from the National Cancer Institute's latest journals.

Martindale's Nursing Centre

http://www.sci.lib.uci.edu/~martindale/Nursing.html

This site is designed to help nurses keep up to date with the latest medical developments. It provides reference material, refresher ideas, and many resources through links such as these: Interactive anatomy browsers, interactive patient browsers, medical dictionaries, nursing courses, nursing references, online nursing journals and more . . .

The Visible Human Project

http://www.nlm.nih.gov/research/visible/visible_human.html

▷ Complete, anatomically detailed, three-dimensional representations of the male and female human body. Transverse CT, MRI and cryosection images of representative cadavers at one millimetre intervals.

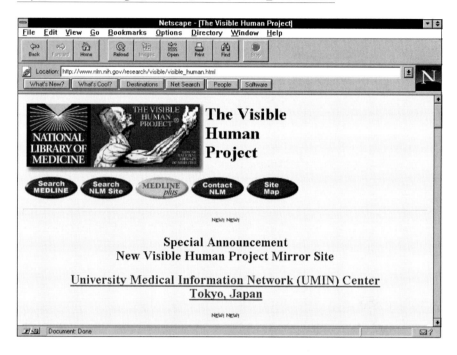

alternative medicine

Alexander Technique, The Complete Guide

http://www.alexandertechnique.com

▷ This is a site that is well worth a visit. Here you will find a systematic guide to Alexander Technique plus other resources – both on and off the Internet.

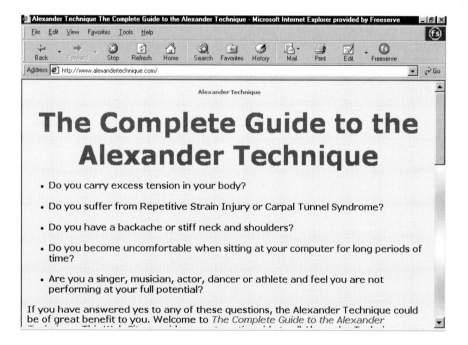

Alternative Medicines Homepage

http://www.pitt.edu/~cbw/altm.html

Therapies here can be classified as unconventional or innovative. Links include information on the following topics: Acupuncture, Chiropractic, Chinese medicine, Medicinal herbs, Osteopathic medicine, Chi, Botanical medicine and many other general alternative medicine resources.

National Oils Research Association Site

http://www.acemake.com/NORA/

A very interesting site to visit.

Natural Medicine, Complementary Health and Alternative Therapies

http://www.teleport.com/

This site is maintained by the Alchemical Medicine Research and Teaching Association. It contains information on cures and alternative therapies taught at US medical schools, health resources, upcoming events in the field, medical and health organisations, and tools for well being.

Aromatherapy

http://www.fragrant.demon.co.uk

This is a guide to Aromatherapy and thousands of links including 600 aromatherapy sites.

general health information

University of Birmingham Department of Nursing

http://www.bham.ac.uk/nursing/

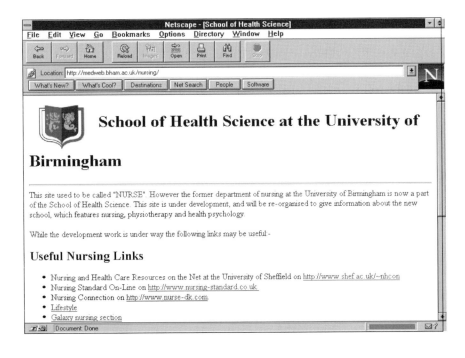

◁ Courses, Internet resources and health-related resource guides.

CYBERNURSE

http://www.cybernurse.com/

If you have an interest in being a nurse or have already taken the plunge, you should find this site useful.

Healthworks Online: Health and Medical Information Service

http://www.healthworks.co.uk

A UK information service.

Martindale's Health Science Guide

http://www.scilib.uci.edu/~martindale/HSGuide.html

Here you will find synopses of teaching files, medical cases, textbooks, courses, images and movies arranged by broad categories such as medical, public health, nutrition and nursing. Very good nursing material.

Medical On-line

http://www.medicalonline.com.au/index.html

This site offers links to the following topics: AIDS information, baby and child, cancer information, contraception and pregnancy, disease index, drugs and drug abuse, health insurance, health yellow pages, medical groups, medical products, nutrition, sex therapy, top ten medical sites, travel health, visible human project and women's health.

Medical/Health Sciences Libraries on the web

http://www.arcade.uiowa.edu/hardin-www/hslibs.html

At this site you will find a meta-index of medical libraries that is organised by state and countries.

NAHAT (National Association of Health Authorities and Trusts)

http://www.nahat.net

Information on the National Health Service and Gateway to the Internet.

Nursing Home Page, University of Iowa

http://indy.radiology.uiowa.ed/Beyond/Nursing/ColOfNurseHP.html

Practising nurses and those aspiring to join the profession will find this site quite useful. It provides information on: College of Nursing homepage, Critical care nursing and Nursing Student homepage.

Nursing Resources on the Internet

http://www.tso.cin.ix.net/user/gl/gloria/nurse.html

Nursing resources and sites; health information; access to nurses' health organisations; access to medical information online and discussion groups.

NHS Glossary

http://www.tcp.co.uk/~iwhc/nhsglss.html

Alphabetical list of terms and abbreviations.

Medweb: Medical Libraries

http://www.MedWeb.Emory.edu/MedWeb

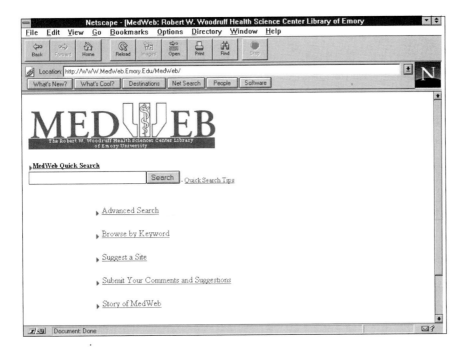

◁ This site contains a list of almost 100 links to medical libraries.

Primary Care Home Page for Nurse Practitioners

http://unhinfo.unh.edu:70/0/unh/acad/health/npract/index.html

This page provides resources related to primary care and other current nursing topics with links such as: Commercial Nursing, Medical Services, Professional News and so on.

Student Nurses' Network

http://www.geocities.com/Athens/4197/nurstat.html

This contains all sorts of information dedicated to the nurses of tomorrow.

UK Directory of Medical and Healthcare Specialists

http://www.ukdirectory.co.uk/com/med.htm

A–Z list of WWW sites.

Virtual Hospital HomePage – University of Iowa

http://vh.radiology.uiowa.edu/

Links to multimedia textbooks and patient information.

OMNI Gateway

http://omni.ac.uk

▷ Outline medical networked information gateway for the UK.

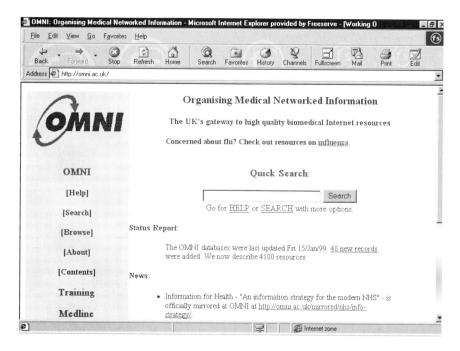

---

mental health nursing, psychiatry and learning disabilities

Internet Mental Health

http://www.mentalhealth.com/p01.html

▷ At this site you will find information on various areas of mental health including:

▷ Internet links
▷ Mental disorders, treatments, and research
▷ Mental health magazine
▷ Psychiatric medications
▷ Publications

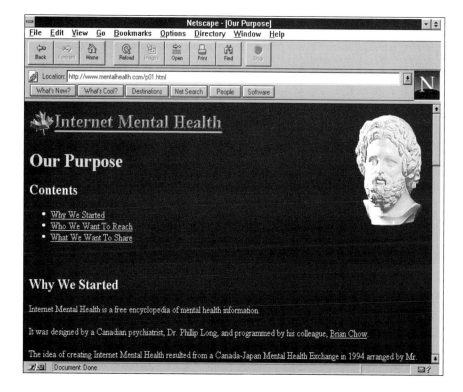

Acorn Care Ltd – Mental Healthcare Nursing – UK

http://www.acorncare.co.uk

This site is maintained by Acorn Care Ltd and provides a forum for discussing issues relating to Mental Health Nursing in the UK, and internationally. Acorn Care staff and other professionals in the sector are encouraged to submit articles and questions.

Centre for Cognitive Therapy

http://www.med.upenn.edu/~psycct/

At this website you will find all sorts of information including frequently asked questions (FAQ) about Cognitive Therapy.

Computers in Mental Health

http://www.ex.ac.uk/cimh/

This is a valuable site to visit. It contains a database of software and other resources.

Cyber-Psych

http://www.charm.net/~pandora/psych/index.html

This site offers lots of information relating to mental health. Some of the resources are: Internet Mental Health Encyclopaedia, mood disorders, Myers-Briggs Personality Profile, national alliance for the mentally ill, psychology and support newsgroups, psychology journals.

Mental Health

http://www.psych.med.uoch.edu/web/aacap

Information from the AACAP, American Academy of Child & Adolescent Psychiatry. Homepage provides links to fact sheets for families.

Mental Health Western Psychiatric Institute and Clinic Library

http://wpic.library.pitt.edu/psychiat.htm

This site has a variety of resources for mental health professionals that link them with other professionals and research. Links include: databases, electronic mental health journals, mental health mailing list, and mental resources by subject and Universities' psychiatric departments.

Hyperguide to MHA 1983

http://www.hyperguide.co.uk/mha

At this site you will find a range of information related to the Mental Health Act 1983.

Mental HealthNet

http://www.cmhcsys.com/mhn.htm

> At this site you will find information on: interactive discussion groups, mental health administration tips, popular articles, self-help resources, tools and information for clinicians.

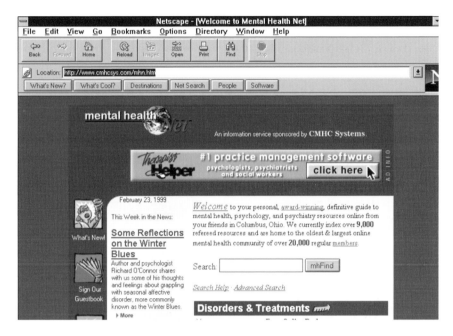

RCN Learning Disability Nurses Forum

http://www.man.ac.uk/LearningDisability/

This is the homepage of The Royal College of Nursing Learning Disability Forum. It is a non commercial site aimed at sharing and developing good practice in Learning Disability. Information is organised under sections such as Conferences, Latest Publications, Useful related sites, News, Forums. You are invited to make contributions to any of the sections.

Disability Net

http://www.disabilitynet.co.uk

Disability Net is described by Paul Matthews as one of the world's leading Internet-based disability information and news services. The site contains a wide variety of information and offers many additional services such as Job Centre (if you are looking for a change in career) and Research (for requesting help with research projects, whether formal or informal).

ARC

http://TheArc.org/welcome.html

The Arc (formerly Association for Retarded Citizens of the United States) is USA's largest voluntary organisation supported by contributions from the general public. The Arc comprises of individuals with mental retardation, family members, professionals in the field of disability and other concerned citizens. It has sections like government report, questions and answers, discussion board and more.

The British Institute of Learning Disabilities

http://www.bild.org.uk/

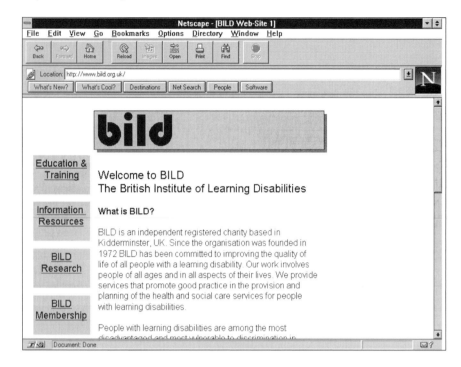

◁ At this site you will find a wide range of information related to learning disability. There is also a section on useful web links, which is quite extensive.

midwifery and health visiting

Women's Health: University of Bristol Dept of O & G

http://www.bris.ac.uk/Depts/ObsGyn

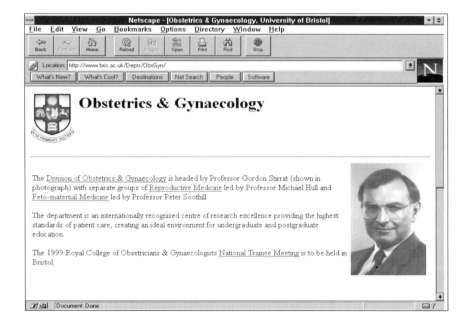

◁ This site should be of value to all health professionals with special interest in obstetrics and gynaecology. Here you will find reproductive medicine websites for:

▷ British Fertility Society
▷ British Andrology Society
▷ Virtual Ovarian Workshop
▷ Society for Low Temperature Biology

Guide to Women's Health Issues

http://asa.ugl.lib.umich.edu/chdocs/womenhealth/toc.html

This site offers information on general health resources and emotional, physical and sexual health topics.

Nursing Web Servers

http://www-son.hs.washington.ed/www-servers.html

This site has some good general nursing references as well as specialised resources. For example: Midwifery List, Oncology Net, Trauma info pages, Women's Health site.

Women's Health Resources on the Internet

http://asa.ugl.lib.umich.edu:80/chdocs/womenhealth/womens_health.html

This site focuses on health issues that are of special interest to women and includes the following links:

- Emotional health topics such as body image/eating disorders, relationships, and stress management;
- Physical health issues such as fitness, nutrition, and gynaecological exams;
- Sexual health issues such as pregnancy, menopause, and birth control.

Online Birth Centre

http://www.efn.org/~djz/birth/birthindex.html

Midwifery, pregnancy and birth-related information.

paediatric nursing and medicine

Pediatric Points of Interest

http://www.med.jhu.edu/peds/neonatology/

▷ Here you will find a searchable collection of links to resources in Paediatrics and Child Health.

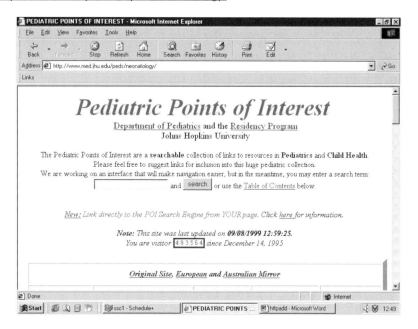

Medical Resources

http://www.ukmedics.com/paediatric.html

At this site you will find information on paediatric assessment and children's health plus several links to other sites of interest such as: children's nursing, Nursing Mothers' Association of Australia, Great Ormond Street Hospital Home Page etc.

Parenting/Child Health Information Database

http://www.cyh.com

This is a really useful site for people working in child health. It has 150 topics about childhood diseases, behaviour and parenting that can easily be printed out and given to parents.

Resources for Nurses and Families

http://pegasus.cc.ucf.edu/~wink/home.html

Here is a site where you will find teaching resources, Internet search engines, Internet resources and much more.

Visible Embryo

http://www.visembryo.com/baby/index.html

This is an interesting site. You will be able to see the embryo at each stage of development and it also contains other materials including a quiz to keep you on your toes.

paramedical

Pharmaceutical Information Network

http://www.pharminfo.com

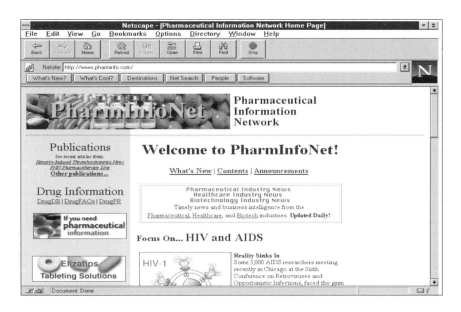

◁ Both patients and health care professionals will find the databases of disease and drugs located at this site quite useful. There is also information about medical science bulletins and other pharmacy links.

RX List

http://www.rxlist.com/

The Internet drug index. Search for a drug name or pull up the top 200 drugs by brand name, manufacturer and generic name.

The Nutrition Expert

http://www.alaska.net/~tne/

This site provides information on the following: cholesterol, diabetes control, eating disorders, health food, sports nutrition, and weight loss.

The Virtual Dental Centre

http://www.sci.lib.uci.edu:80/~martindale/Dental.html

This site offers information that will help you improve your chances about preventative dental care.

The Site for Student Radiographers and Schools

http://www.soft.net.uk/nold

This is a site designed for students. Take a look and see what you think.

MUSC – Occupational Therapy Home

http://www.musc.edu/chp-rehab/ot/othome.htm

This page is being developed as a comprehensive resource for information regarding the MUSC program, events relating to OT in South Carolina, and resources that would be valuable to occupational therapists everywhere.

healthcare research

British Medical Journal (BMJ)

http://www.bmj.com/index.shtml

▷ This site, among other things, contains the full text of all articles published in the weekly *BMJ* from Jan 1996. Access to the entire site is free.

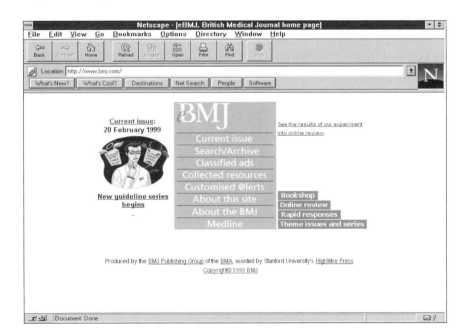

Cardiac Prevention Research Centre

http://www.ccn.cs.dal.ca/Health/CPRC/home_pg.html

This site offers information on coronary heart disease.

Nightingale Nursing Resources

http://nightingale.con.utl.edu/

At this site you can use the search features or select a high-level link that leads to more detailed breakdowns by topic. First-level selections include these categories: education, practice, professional nursing communications, publications, research and more.

Nurse (Warwick University)

http://www.medweb.bham.ac.uk/nursing/

A searchable nursing information service. This contains links to other services for nurses, nursing sites, a midwife page, papers and journals, contacts for nurses with special interests, institutions with e-mail addresses, jobs, nursing and health-related software packages.

The Cochrane Collaboration

http://hiru.mcmaster.ca/cochrane/

The Cochrane Collaboration is an international not-for-profit organisation. At this site you should find up-to-date, accurate information about the effects of healthcare. Reviews are prepared mostly by healthcare professionals who volunteer to work in one of more than 40 Collaborative Review Groups.

Netting the Evidence

http://www.shef.ac.uk/academic/R-Z/scharr/ir/netting.html

"Netting the Evidence" is a very useful resource. It is a SCHARR introduction to Evidence Based Practice on the Internet. Well worth a visit.

Evidence Based Practice for Mental Health and Learning Disability

http://www.psychiatry.ox.ac.uk/oxamweb/

This is an Evidence Based Practice web resource for mental health and learning disability.

Digest of Health Related Research Funding and Training Opportunities
http://www.leeds.ac.uk/rdinfo/

▷ Here you will find a selected list of Major Funding Sources. The list is regularly updated and contains those sources that are most likely to be relevant. However, there is a list of other funding organisations with limited information.

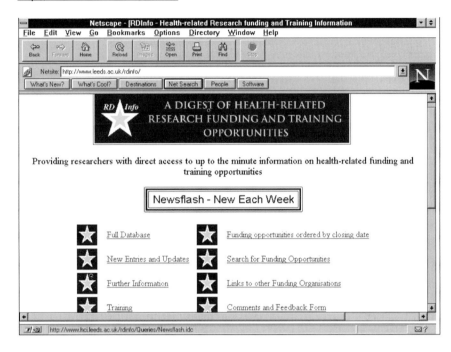

journals for health professionals

RCN Nursing Standard Online
http://www.nursing-standard.co.uk

▷ At this web site you will find a selection of articles and abstracts from the weekly issue of *Nursing Standard*, plus details of conferences and continuing education opportunities.

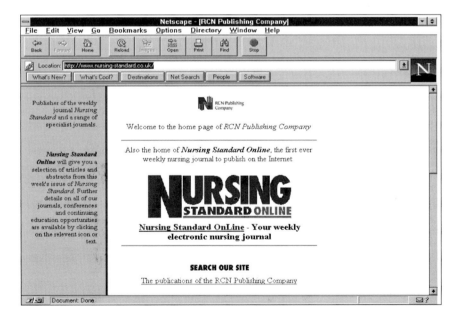

Health Service Journal (HSJ)

http://www.hsj.co.uk

The HSJ online is the UK's leading health policy and management web site. It is the interactive version of Health Service Journal. It has an average of 100,000 page impressions per week. At present the information provided on HSJ online is free. Recently included is a section called HSJ Jobs Plus which carries all job adverts that have appeared in the Health Service Journal. You can search for jobs according to category and location and respond immediately via e-mail. HSJ Jobs Plus also includes an extensive training section and details of the latest NHS tenders.

BMJ

http://www.bmj.com/bmj/bmjpubs/sites.htm

This is a selection of WWW sites of medical interest.

Evidence-Based Nursing

http://www.bmjpg.com/data/ebn.htm

This is a new high quality international journal. It gives you access to the best research related to nursing and keeps you up to date with the most important new evidence within nursing. Expert commentators have put every article into a clinical context and draw out the key research findings. From this site you will find a link to the *Nursing Standard* online website.

libraries and free health databases

Healthworks Online

http://www.healthworks.co.uk

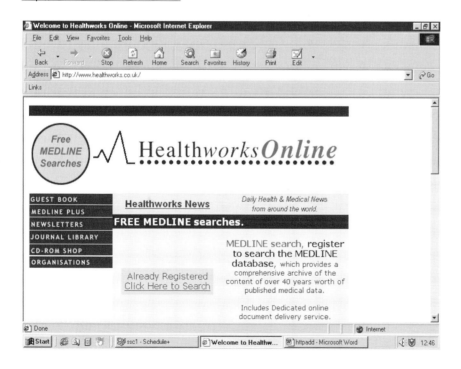

◁ Here you will have free access to Medline from home, college or any Internet connected PC with unlimited searches.

Emergency Nursing on the Internet

http://www.Emergency-Nurse.com

Accident and Emergency Online has now been relaunched and is the home of A&E nursing on the Internet. Here you can search a selection of databases such as Medline, Toxline, Aidsline and Cancerlit. The databases are offered free of charge and no password or username is required to enter the site. New features include: Course and Conference calender, an articles & abstracts section, and more nursing humour. The existing sections have been improved and updated. There are now over 150 Emergency Nursing contacts in the e-directory, details on UK pay scales, information on the new UK nursing newsgroup 'uk-sci.med.nursing', and lots more.

HENSA

http://www.hensa.ac.uk

This is a national service that benefits the Higher Education and Research Community in the UK. It maintains copies of electronic archives from all over the world, providing access to a wide range of up-to-date software and other material which is available free of charge to anyone from the UK HE Community.

Internet Public Library

http://www.ipl.org

This is the first public library of and for the Internet community. When you visit this site you will find a useful section called FAQs where you will find the answers to all your questions about this site.

NHS IM&T Electronic Library

http://www.ctf.imc.exec.nhs.uk/

This is an online knowledge base for all involved in the management and delivery of Information Management and Technology (IM&T) within the English NHS. You will be able to browse or search the electronic library and much more.

Open Software Library (OSL)

http://www.personal.u-net.com/~osl/

OSL publishes and distributes education and training material for nurses and other health professionals. Here you will find software on CD-ROMs, disks and videos covering a wide spectrum of nursing and healthcare education.

PubMed

http://www.ncbi.nlm.nih/gov/PubMed

UKOLN

http://road/ukoln.ac.uk/cgi-bin/egwcgi.egwirtcl/mmed.egw

National Board Health Care Database

http://www.enb.org.uk/hcd.htm

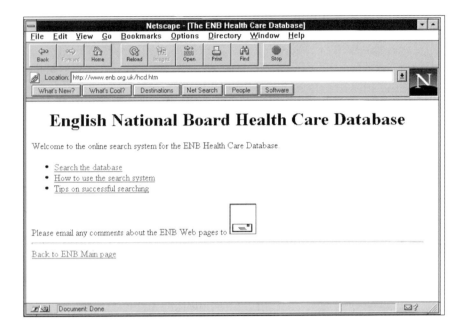

◁ At this site you will find an online search system. You can search the database for health related information. Information on how to use the search system and tips on successful searching are provided.

electronic publication and citation

Citing Internet Resources

http://www.eeicom.com/eye/utw/96aug.html

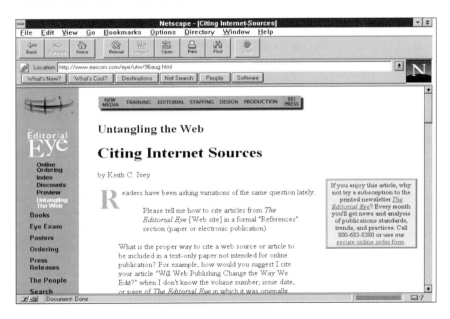

◁ The "Eye" is a resource for anyone who cares about con-temporary publishing practices. Any aspect of effective printed, electronic, visual or spoken communication is likely to appear as a topic in the Eye. At this site, students of health studies will find several useful articles including help on the proper way to cite web resources.

Citation of Digital Publishing

http://www.uvm.ed/~xli/reference/apa.html

Citing Electronic Resources

http://www.ipl.org/ref/QUE/FARQ/netcite/FARQ.html

Internet Publishing
http://www.sscnet.ucla.edu/ssc/franks/book/

This is the HTML version of the "Internet Publishing Handbook for World-Wide Web, Gopher, and WAIS by Mike Franks". It is complete with publication data, dedication, acknowledgements, a collection of Internet links (URLs) from the book, and a note on differences between the HTML and printed versions of this book. The paper version is available in bookstores.

quality of public services

Lasernet: The 'Service First' Quality Network for London and the South East
http://www.open.gov.uk/lasernet/index.htm

▷ 'Service First' is a Cabinet Office Unit of the British Government and a principle underpinning the delivery of all public services.

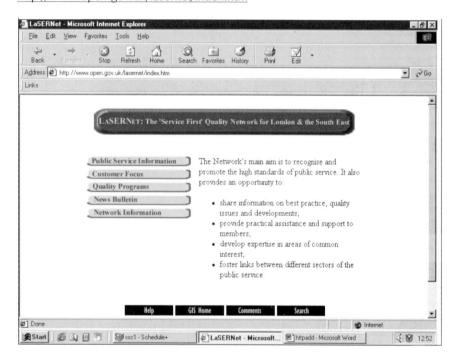

I hope you have managed to access all the sites listed above and you have found some, if not all, of them useful. Some web sites are updated more often than others. New ones are appearing all the time, while others vanish in thin air. As you get attached to the Net you may want to look at new sites. No problem! Just pay a visit to Rod Ward's web page: Nursing & Healthcare Resources on the Net at:

http://www.shef.ac.uk/~nhcon

Here you will find a list of over 1000 nursing and related web sites with a UK bias.

summary and conclusion

With the help of a suitable browser such Internet Explorer or NetScape Navigator or Communicator you can surf through the net jumping from place to place in computer databases all over the world by using the hypertext links. You can also browse through the net by using URLs you know about, or try the ones listed in this Unit. Do remember that the Net is constantly changing. Therefore when you encounter an address to which you cannot connect, try connecting to the host system without specifying a specific document.

finding health information on the internet

"Searching the Internet for specific information is a daunting prospect for most of us, rather like being presented with the task of finding a very small fly in a very large web!" *Howson (1997)[2]*

Information Officer,
ScHARR – University of Sheffield
e-mail: n.j.howson@sheffield.ac.uk

With so much information in Cyberspace, you may wonder where you should start to find the health information you want. Wonder no more. There are people out there who have created tools that you can use to make it easy for you to find what you are looking for. In this unit you will be introduced to a few valuable tools that are ridiculously easy to use. You will get to meet two other inhabitants of the Net: Information Gateways and *online* **Databases**. You will also have an opportunity to explore specific databases using effective search strategies to find information for your projects.

> **TECHNO TALK**
>
> A <u>database</u> can be described as a sophisticated electronic filing cabinet capable of storing and sorting large amounts of data in an organised manner. The data can be accessed quickly.

checklist

Below is a checklist of what you can expect to find out in this Unit. Read through
the statements then tick (✓) the items about which you would like to know more.

I would like to find out more about:

Please turn over the page and read through the topics you have ticked

Although there are millions of web pages in cyberspace, **Web Directories** and **Search Engines** are two valuable tools that will help you find materials on the Web. They are designed to help you navigate the Internet quickly and efficiently. There are various species of Web directories and Search engines. The number is growing all the time.

4.1.1 web directories

Web Directories, unlike Search Engines, are created by humans (rather than robots), and organise Web pages into various categories, sometimes with reviews and ratings of web sites. Table 4.1 outlines three of the best.

table 4.1

POPULAR WEB DIRECTORIES	
Yahoo! UK & Ireland	http://www.yahoo.co.uk Yahoo has been around since 1994. According to recent evaluations and studies, Yahoo is the best subject tree to start with and the one that has consistently been found to be both useful and fun. It is a searchable, browsable hierarchical index of the Internet. 'Yahoo' highlights listings that are about or of particular interest to Web users in the UK, Ireland and the expatriate community. Its coverage is general, but searching and browsing can be limited to health topics.
Achoo	http://www.achoo.com/ This is a health focus version of Yahoo covering approximately 7,000 indexed and searchable sites. It has three main categories: practice of medicine, human life and the business of health. Although there is a searching facility, browsing the index is a better option. An updated and improved version is under development, to include better searching facilities.
InfoSeek Select Sites	http://guide.infoseek.com/ This search engine has several categories including Health and Medicine.
Magellan	http://www.mckinley.com/ This search engine includes categories such as Communications, Daily Living, Food, Health, Humanities, Science, Law, Environment, and Spirituality.

4.1.1.1 carrying out a search using a web directory

Most Search tools tend to be biased towards the United States. It may be worthwhile to start our first activity in this section with a tool that is very easy to use and that allows us to limit to just the United Kingdom. For this reason I have picked Yahoo – but it is important to bear in mind that most web directories work in the same way, and also look much the same.

Suppose we wanted to find some information on a particular medical condition, let's say *Meningitis.* We can ask Yahoo to use this keyword to search its entire database and offer a list of sites containing information on this medical condition.

For hands-on experience, carry out the steps listed in **Worksheet 5**. When you are done, please return to this section and read on.

When you have completed the activity turn to the next page and read on

SEARCHING WITH YAHOO'S WEB DIRECTORY　　worksheet **5**

1 Log on to Windows.

2 Start your browser.

3 Enter the following URL in the location box
http://www.yahoo.co.uk

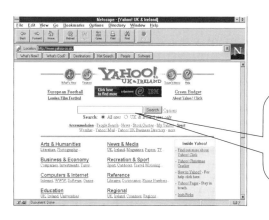

4 Point and click in this textbox. A flashing cursor should appear.

NOTE

When you arrive at the Yahoo site you will see a page like the one shown in the screenshot. You will notice it has a search-engine style textbox into which you can type keywords. Since we know exactly what we are looking for (ie, information on meningitis), we can use this textbox to do a search.

5 Type the keyword: **meningitis**, then click the Search button. *After a few seconds you should see a new page listing the sites that matched your search criteria.*

6 Click on any of the links that interest you. If the page does not interest you, click on the **Back** button on your browser's toolbar to return to the search results and try a different one. When you have had enough, click on **Home** button on the toolbar.

Sometimes you may want to search for something that can't be encapsulated in a single word, in these cases you can use the following strategies, which most search engines and web directories will understand (and those that don't will generally ignore them).

- You can enter several keywords, type the most important keyword followed by the least important. For example, if you wanted to find 'research studies in nursing', type **nursing research**. This list will present good links to nursing sites before the rather more general links to sites, which only contain research studies.

- Use uppercase characters only if you expect to find uppercase characters. Searching for 'DISEASE' may find very little, searching for 'Disease' should find a lot.

- To find a particular phrase, enclose it in "quote marks". For example, a search for "Anorexia Nervosa" would find only pages containing this phrase and ignore pages that just contain one word or the other.

- Prefix a word with a '+' sign if it must be included, and with a '-' sign if it must be excluded. For example, if you're searching for Insomnia in men, you could type **+insomnia men –women**. Similarly, you could type tumours **–benign** to ensure that you did not find pages about benign tumours.

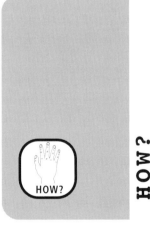

HOW?

How to set search options

Yahoo! UK & Ireland will normally search categories, titles, and comments to find listings that contain all of your keywords. Equally, Yahoo! will not pay attention to case (eg, "National Meningitis Trusts" is treated just like "national meningitis trusts") and will stop after it finds 100 matches. However, you can customise your search. You can specify:

- whether you want matches to contain all of your keywords or at least one of your keywords;

- whether your keywords should be considered as substrings or whole words;

- the number of matches displayed per page.

4.1.1.3 search results

Yahoo! searches retrieve the following three different kinds of information:

- Categories that match your keywords;
- Web sites that match your keywords;
- Categories where those sites are listed.

Thus, you can choose to go directly to retrieve sites, or browse around relevant categories for related information.

4.1.1.4 browsing yahoo's web directory

While carrying out the previous activity, you may have noticed that below the Yahoo textbox into which you typed your keywords, there were a collection of hypertext links offering broad categories which you can use to dig deeper to find more specific information (see Figure 4.1).

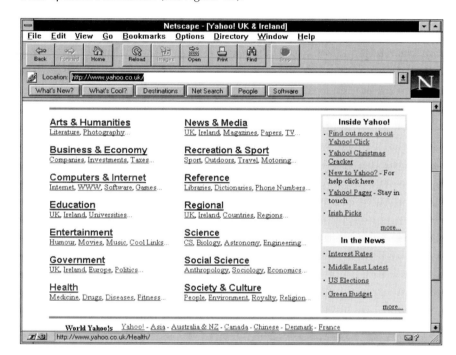

◁ fig 4.1 **Hypertext links**

A list of hypertext links offering broad categories, which can be used to dig deeper for more specific information.

When you carry out the activity below, you would no doubt discover how easy it is to follow the Yahoo layout. Yahoo has used **bold** and plain text to help you navigate intelligently. Bold text means this is a link to another Yahoo category; plain text indicates that it's a link to a page elsewhere on the Web that contains the kind of information you have been searching for.

BROWSING YAHOO! UK & IRELAND   activity **4.2**

In the previous activity we had a particular Internet site in mind. We were looking for sites dealing with a medical condition called meningitis. Since we knew exactly what we wanted we were able to use the Search facility. But what if we did not have a particular Internet site in mind? In such a case we could have used the Browse facility to 'surf' the Net and see what is there. To do this, we simply point and click on a topic we want to browse.

Before reading on, it is suggested that you carry out the steps listed in **Worksheet 6**.

When you have completed the activity return to p. 78 and read on

① If you are not logged on, re-start your browser and . . .

② Enter the following URL in the Location/Address box
http://www.yahoo.co.uk

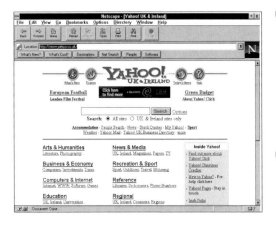

③ Point and click on the category 'Health'. (If you can't see it, use the scrollbar to move down.) *A new page should appear displaying a list of subcategories.*

④ Now, point and click on any sub-category of your choice. *This should move you to yet another page.*

⑤ If the page does not interest you, click on the **Back** button on your browser's toolbar to return to the sub-category list and try a different one. When you have had enough, click on **Home** button on the toolbar.

NOTE

In the previous activity, we knew exactly what we were looking for. In this activity we know exactly what we are looking for. Therefore, we can select a broad category and dig deeper.

Take a look at the screen shot in Fig. 4.2. You should be able to see a number in brackets next to each of the categories. You may have already encountered this feature and wondered what it means. This number tells you how many links you can expect to find in that category. For example, in the category *Diseases and Conditions* I found 5573 links.

▷ fig 4.2 **Browsing**

The screenshot on the right shows sub-headings with number of links in brackets.

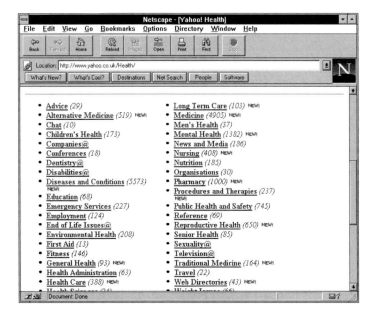

4.1.2 search engines

When you start your Browser (eg, NetScape Navigator), you should see a range of Search engines. The number is growing. Table 4.2 lists the most popular ones. When using search engines, you will make your search a little easier if you consider the keywords, synonyms and phrases that might help the search. For more Searching Tips, pay a visit to:

http://www.wfi.fr/volterre/searchtips.html

table 4.2

POPULAR SEARCH ENGINES	
Medical World Search	http://www.mwsearch.com/ This search engine was especially developed for the medical field. It indexes the full content of the major medical sites on the web, enabling users to search for any word in any of the pages indexed. It supports the use of Boolean operators: AND and OR. It allows for phrase and word group searching. Once a search is complete, a list of related and more specific words appear, at this point you can change your search using Boolean operators and terms from the thesaurus. For example, typing the keyword 'disease' produces 34147 documents, entering the keyword 'diseases in twins, (a thesaurus term) produces a more precise two documents.
Lycos	http://www.lycos.com This is one of the biggest search engines. It claims to have indexed 91 per cent of the Web. The index searches by document title, links and keywords. It offers many search options and returns a ranked list with options for terse or long display. It is often busy.
HotBot	http://www.hotbot.com This is a highly recommended search engine. It has over 54 million documents.
AltaVista	http://www.altavista.digital.com This search engine has over 8 billion words covering over 30 million web pages. For tips on searching with AltaVista, visit Roy Bowers Webpage at http://www.tnis.net/rbowers/search.html
Excite	http://www.excite.com This search engine has full text to over 11.5 million pages and is updated weekly.
InfoSeek	http://www.infoseek.com InfoSeek has been voted by *PC Computing* magazine's editors as the most valuable search tool for 1995. It allows for phrase searching, which greatly increases the quality of your results. It also has a guide to the "best of the Web".
InfoSeek Ultra	http://ultra.infoseek.com This new search engine from InfoSeek is fast and furious.
WebCrawler	http://www.webcrawler.com This search engine is fast, relatively easy to use, indexes titles, as well as content, recently absorbed by America Online and returns a ranked list of hits with no descriptions. It includes a list of the 25 most visited sites on the web.

Until recently the best search tools were available free of charge. Since some of them now require a subscription fee, some of the tools listed above may not be available for you to use on your college computer network.

How to select the right search engine to use

Deciding which one to choose is difficult, as there is no known single search tool that can satisfy every query. However, connection difficulties will often make this choice for you. As you start using these tools you will soon find out that Lycos is rarely available during work hours. Webcrawler is more often available, is easy to use, and as a consequence will often be your first choice. InfoSeek has been favourably reviewed and rated number one in several recent studies. Excite and the others are also worth exploring. Here are a few points to bear in mind:

▷ Different search engines offer different search options. The available search options are usually detailed in help pages associated with each search engine.

▷ Different search engines are better for some searches than others. For example, WebCrawler is an inappropriate tool for an author or name search, but its full page indexing can be very effective when looking for an obscure term.

▷ Webcrawler indexes every word of a Web page, while the Lycos index is built with only selected words, such as the title, the headings, and the most significant 100 words. These differences contribute to the very different result sets that are returned by different search engines for the same query.

HOW?

HOW?

4.1.2.1 carrying out a search using a search engine

Most search engines look much the same and more or less work in the same way. For our next activity let's use Lycos. When you run Lycos, you'll see a page similar to the one shown in the screenshot below (Fig. 4.3).

▷ fig. 4.3 **The Lycos Homepage**

This is the starting page for Lycos. To search the web, simply type your keyword or keywords in the textbox and then press the Enter key on your keyboard.

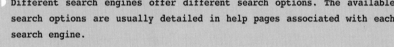

After you have typed a keyword (or keywords) into the textbox, press the **Enter** key on your keyboard. Your browser will send the information off to the engine.

EXPLORING A WEB SITE USING LYCOS   activity **4.3**

To compare Lycos with Yahoo, let's us once again attempt to find information on the medical condition meningitis.

For hands-on experience, follow the steps listed in **Worksheet 7**.

When you have completed the activity return to the next page and read on

SEARCHING WITH LYCOS   worksheet **7**

① Log On to Windows and start your browser.

② Enter the following URL in the Location/Address box
http://www.lycos.com

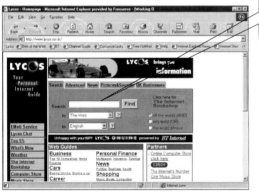

③ Point and click in this textbox. *A flashing cursor should appear.*

④ Type the keyword: **meningitis**, then click the **Find** button. *After a few seconds you should see a new page listing the sites that matched your search criteria.*

> **NOTE**
>
> When you arrive at the Lycos site you will see a page like the one shown in the screenshot. You will notice it is not so dissimilar to Yahoo. It has a search-engine textbox into which you can type keywords. Since we know exactly what you are looking for (ie, information on meningitis), we can use this textbox to do a search.

⑤ Click on any of the links that interest you. If the page does not interest you, click on the **Back** button on your browser's toolbar to return to the search results and try a different one. When you have had enough, click on **Home** button on the toolbar.

Once Lycos has found the sites that matched your search criteria, it lists the first ten. (To see all ten matches you may need to use the scroll bar to expose the parts that are hidden at the bottom of the screen.) Once you have looked at the first ten you can go to the next ten, then the next and so on. If you have followed a link and you are not satisfied with the content you can go back. Just click on the **Back** button on the browser's toolbar.

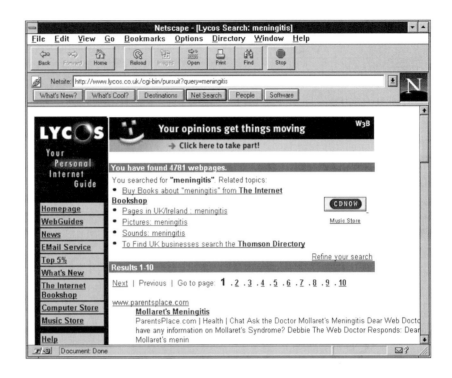

> fig. 4.4 **Search Criteria**

An ill-defined search could result in 100s of sites being identified – most of which may not be relevant. For example, as shown in the screenshot on the right, a search on the keyword 'meningitis' found 4781 related web pages.

If you find that too many sites have been identified, it is most likely that you have not defined your search criteria well enough. You should try again using more specific keywords or keyphrases.

Some search engines give the pages a score for relevancy. As a rule of thumb you should only consider pages with a score of 75% or above. If you can't find what you are looking for with one search engine, always try another. Different search engines use different methods of searching and can produce different results. To experience the differences do the next activity.

activity 4.4 EXPLORING A WEB SITE USING ALTERNATIVE SEARCH ENGINES

Now carry out a few searches using the other Search engines listed in Table 4.2 (p. 78).

When you have completed the activity return to this page and read on

If after completing this section you still feel you need more help on using Search Engines, pay a visit to this Web site:

http://daphne.palomar.edu/TGSEARCH

4.2 information gateways for health and medical sources

Anyone can publish on the Net. It is, therefore, unsurprising that the Internet is packed with all sorts of information. The down side is that as there is no quality control, most of the available information has not been evaluated. To deal with the problems of quality and quantity, Information **Gateways** have been developed. Some of these gateways have been funded by Higher Education in the United Kingdom to provide a filtering service for Internet resources. Having completed the activities in the previous section you will have identified how many hits you found when searching for the medical condition: 'Viral Meningitis'.

Information Gateways are different from search engines, as they are more like an online catalogue for the Internet; ie, they will only have details of the very best web links in a particular subject. The process of filtering is carried out by a team of experts employed for that purpose. Since exploring the Internet is rather like diving into an electronic boot fair, the information gateways can be a very useful starting point. As a student of healthcare you should find these three information gateways quite useful: NHS gateway, OMNI and SOSIG (pronounced sausage).

4.2.1 nhs gateway (medical and nhs resources)

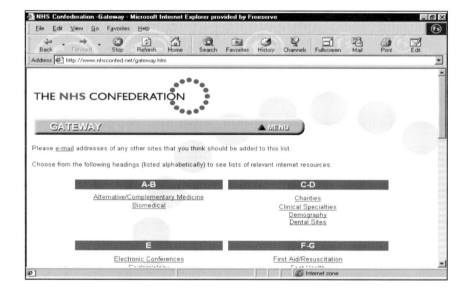

◁ fig. 4.5 **The NHS gateway**

To access NHS gateway, enter this URL in the Location/address box of your browser:

http://www.nhsconfed.net/gateway.htm

When you reach the NHS gateway homepage you can choose relevant Internet resources from a series of headings arranged alphabetically. Table 4.3 shows the possibilities:

table 4.3

A–B

Alternative/Complementary Medicine
Biomedical

C–D

Charities
Clinical Specialities
Demography
Dental Sites

E

Electronic Conferences
Epidemiology
Evidence Based Healthcare

F–G

First Aid/Resuscitation
Foot Health
General Practice
Government – National & Global

H

Health Economics
Health Promotion and Preventative
   Healthcare
Healthcare Informatics Specialist Groups
Healthcare Management
Hospice
HyperGuide to the Mental Health Act

I–L

Information Technology for Health
   Professionals
Jobs
Journals
Laboratories
Learning Resources
Lewingtons Mental Health Article
Libraries
Locality Commissioning

M–N

Mental Health
News
NHS Community Health Councils
NHS Executive
NHS Health Authorities
NHS Health Boards
NHS Press Releases
NHS Special Authorities
NHS Trusts
Nursing Site

O–P

Occupational & Environmental
Other Health Related Sites
Patient Information
Pharmaceutical
Primary Care
Professional Allied to Medicine
Professional and Management Groups
Public Health
Purchasing

R

Research Councils
Research Networks
Royal Colleges

S–U

Services to the NHS
UK Medical Schools

4.2.2 omni

OMNI (Organising Medical Networked Information) is another gateway to high quality Internet resources in medicine, biomedicine, allied health, health management and related topics. It provides comprehensive coverage of the UK resources in this area and access to the best resources worldwide. Using a process of selection, evaluation and description the collection is continuously being updated. The OMNI databases were last updated Fri 15/Jan/99 and at that point 4100 resources were described.

To use OMNI simply enter this URL in the Location/Address box of your browser:

http://omni.ac.uk/

A page like the screenshot below should appear. Enter appropriate keyword(s) in the 'Quick Search' box, and click the search button.

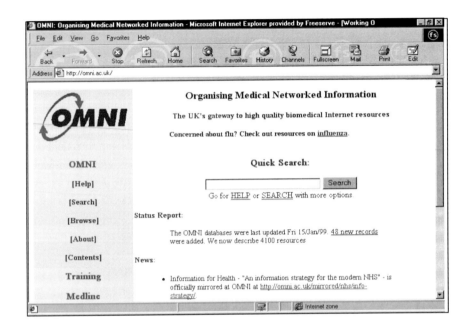

◁ fig. 4.6 **The OMNI homepage**

4.2.3 sosig

SOSIG (short for Social Science Information Gateway – was the first subject-based information gateway in the United Kingdom and established in 1994. It contains approximately 5000 high quality information resources for social scientists to use. The Internet resources cover a range of different formats from books, reports, newsletters, bibliographies, databases, mailing lists and software. Table 4.4 below lists the range of subjects covered by SOSIG.

table 4.4

THE RANGE OF SUBJECTS COVERED BY SOSIG	
Demography	Law
Economics, development	Management, Accountancy, Business
Education	Philosophy
Environmental Issues	Politics – International Relations
Ethnology, Social Anthropology	Psychology
Feminism	Social Science, General Methodology
Geography	Social Welfare Community Disability
Government, Military Science	Sociology
	Statistics – Demography

The SOSIG Internet Catalogue is structured in a way that allows you either to browse resource descriptions within subject headings or to use keyword searching of the descriptions. The SOSIG button bar is available at the top of every page and will help you navigate through the Gateway. To use SOSIG visit this URL:

http://www.sosig.ac.uk

4.2.3 health on the net (hon)

This is very similar to OMNI. The database has been created manually. Contents of each site have been reviewed and supplemented by an automatically generated database. But, unlike OMNI, searching is automatically carried out across both databases. Search results are placed into two categories: reviewed and unreviewed. It permits simple and advanced searching (Boolean operators, wildcards, phrase searching). In addition you will find a searchable database of medical images and movies, selected abstracts and full text papers from conferences and journals and information about conferences and events. To use this HON type this URL in the Location/Address box of your browser:

http:/www.hon.ch/

activity 4.5 BOOKMARKING SITES OF INTEREST

- Visit the NHS Gateway. At the homepage select from the list offered a heading that interests you.
- Add NHS Gateway to your bookmark list. (For Help refer to Section 3.2.3 and Worksheet 4.)
- Visit the SOSIG gateway and browse the resource descriptions within the subject headings.
- Add SOSIG Gateway to your bookmark list.
- Visit the HON gateway and browse the resource descriptions within the subject headings.
- Add HON Gateway to your hotlist.

DATABASE SEARCHING USING OMNI

Carry out the task set in **Worksheet 8**. You will find step-by-step instructions on how to carry out a basic search on OMNI.

When you have completed the activity return to the next page and read on

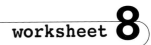
① Log On to Windows and start your browser.

② Enter the following URL in the Location/Address box
http://omni.ac.uk

③ Point and click in the command **Browse**. *A long list of categories should appear.*

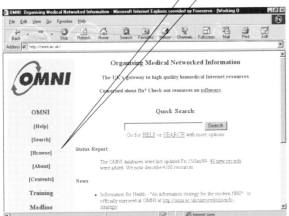

④ Select **Nursing**.

⑤ Select **ENB healthcare database**.

⑥ Read what the description says.

⑦ Click on the **heading** or **URL**.

⑧ Add the **ENB healthcare database** to your hotlist.

This section has introduced you to the world of subject-based information gateways, which you can use to navigate the Information Superhighway, in the same way you might use a road map. It won't feature all the byways and side roads of the Internet, but will serve you as a basic navigational guide.

4.3 online databases relevant to health students and staff

The range of *databases* available to health students and staff has grown at an alarming rate. To provide a detailed explanation of each is beyond the scope of this unit. Some of the possibilities are: CINAHL (Cumulative Index of Nursing and Allied Health Literature) and Medline. Both of these databases are important resources to help you keep up-to-date with new developments in health literature.

CINAHL and Medline are usually described as bibliographic databases as the records on these databases are mostly just references to published material. The most common publication types are articles published in professional/academic journals. However the trend is for some databases to include access to full-text material, distinct from just the reference.

Here are two examples of how a record on a bibliographic database might look like. The first example is a record of a published book, and the second example is a record of a published journal article.

EXAMPLE 1	A RECORD OF A PUBLISHED BOOK
Accessions no.	007
Author's name	Chellen, S.S.
Book title	Information Technology for the Caring Professions: a user's handbook
Publisher	Cassell
Publication year	1995
Publication type	Book
Subject heading 1	Computers, Nursing
Subject heading 2	History of Computing
Subject heading 3	Information Technology

EXAMPLE 2	A RECORD OF A PUBLISHED JOURNAL ARTICLE
Accessions no.	008
Author's name	Chellen, S.S.
Article title	A Layman's Guide to IT
Publisher	Occupational Health: a Journal for Occupational Health Nurses 47 (10), 351-2, 354-5
Publication year	1995
Publication type	Journal article
Subject heading 1	Occupational Health
Subject heading 2	Information Technology
Subject heading 3	Databases
Subject heading 4	Computers

Each line indicated in the above records represents a different sort of information, ie, *accession number, author's name, title, publisher, date of publication, type of publication* and *subject headings*. Each line (aspect) is called a field. So you can see from the previous tables that both publications have the year 1995 in the field labelled 'Publication Year'.

Imagine you were doing a search on a database that contains the two records shown above. If you type in the Search box the keyword ***Information Technology***, both records will be found because both have a field with the words Information Technology recorded. However, if you were to type the keyword ***Databases***, only the journal article would be found as there is no specific mention of databases in the record for the book by Sydney Chellen.

On CINAHL and Medline subject headings, which are added to the records, enhance the reference by describing accurately what it is about. The choice of subject headings will vary from database to database. For example, one health database may use the term Old Age, another may use the term Aged. Therefore to do a search for Elderly is not likely to be as successful, in terms of records found. How do you know then?

Some database services will map your term to the best subject headings on the database relevant. This allows some assistance to you when searching, as it will help to format the search strategy. Otherwise it is a good idea to be thinking laterally about your search, ie, thinking of alternative words or expressions to use when searching a subject.

With the development of compact discs the trend in the information world was to store databases on compact discs called CD-ROMS. Since the escalation of the use of the Internet, a range of commercial databases, increasingly with full-text services, is becoming available through this channel. One of the leading electronic information retrieval services is Ovid Technologies Inc. CINAHL and Medline are just two examples of databases that were only available on CD-ROM, but now have become available on the Net. (For more information see Unit 1 – under the heading: Databases).

There are advantages and limitations with every database so it is practical to become competent with a number of different search tools when researching a subject. There are still benefits in adopting the traditional hand searching of the journals literature. This is especially important with the latest copies of a journal title. Remember it can be several months before a reference published in a journal will be available on a bibliographic database and even then not everything which is published in any particular journal issue would end up on a database.

WHAT'S AVAILABLE?   activity **4.6**

Although more and more electronic databases are becoming available for use, do not expect to be able to have access to all of them at your local health, college/university or professional library/computing laboratory. Use this checklist to tick (✓) those that are available at your institution and establish if they are on CD-ROMs or part of the Ovid-Biomed service.

○ Medline
○ CINAHL
○ Cancerlit
○ Core Biomedical Collection
○ Ovid Biomedical Collection II, III, IV
○ Mental Health Collection
○ Nursing Collection

When you have completed the activity return to this page and read on

4.3.2 developing search strategies

Most databases allow for the facility to combine terms together using special linking words often called Boolean Operators. These special words (or Boolean Operators) are: AND, OR and NOT. The best way to think of these is to imagine they are like doing equations with words.

table 4.5

BOOLEAN OPERATORS	
AND	Use when you want to limit your search eg, *nursing* and *stress*
	(Limits search to references on nursing and stress, i.e. both subjects)
OR	Use when you want to broaden your search eg, *nursing* or *midwifery*
	(Broadens search to include all articles on nursing and all articles on midwifery, ie, not necessarily in the same reference)
NOT	Use when you want to limit your search eg, *nursing* not *midwifery*
	(Limits your search by removing references to a subject you are not interested in)

activity **4.7** WRITING A SEARCH STATEMENT

You have been given a task to research the truth about waiting lists in NHS Hospitals.

▷ Identify what are the keywords or keyphrases you will have to look up on any database, such as CINAHL or Medline. Write them down on a piece of paper.
▷ Now try writing a search statement using the Boolean Operators discussed in Section 4.3.2 and the keywords/keyphrases you have identified.

When you have completed the activity return to this page and read on

4.3.3 searching databases

This final section gives you the opportunity to put into practice some of the things you have been learning about in this Unit. Following Activity 4.7, you should now know what health databases are available to you in your local health, college or professional library. If you are searching the Internet from home here are four free databases that you should be able to use for the next activity. For advice I strongly suggest you consult your librarian.

▷ ENB Healthcare Database
http://www.enb.org.uk/hcd.htm

▷ PubMed
http://www.ncbi.nlm.nih/gov/PubMed

▶ UKOLN
http://roads/ukoln.ac.uk/cgi-bin/egwcgi/egwirtcl/mmed.egw

▶ Accident and Emergency Online
http://www.damien.purplenet.co.uk/medline.htm

Remember that navigating your way round the ecology of the Internet will take time but understanding the nature of databases should make it more understandable to you.

SEARCHING HEALTH DATABASES
activity 4.8

1 Question: What clinical guidelines are available for the care of people with asthma?

Task:
▶ Identify keyword(s) or keyphrase(s).
▶ Write out a search statement using Boolean Operators.
▶ Test it out on a database.

2 Question: What does clinical governance mean?

Task:
▶ Identify keyword(s) or keyphrase(s).
▶ Write out a search statement using Boolean Operators.
▶ Test it out on a database.

3 Task:
▶ Think of a subject you would like to research.
▶ Identify keyword(s) or keyphrase(s).
▶ Write out a search statement using Boolean Operators.
▶ Test it out on a database.

4 Task:
BIOMED provides access to a range of health databases. These include CINAHL, Medline and collections of fulltext journals. CINAHL is a primary source of bibliographical information for Nursing and Midwifery literature.

If you have access to the BIOMED service in your institution, complete **Worksheet 9**. It will enable you to search CINAHL more effectively.

When you have completed the activity return to p. 100 and read on

PART ONE

NOTE

CINAHL is a primary source of bibliographical information for Nursing and Midwifery literature. This Worksheet is divided in four parts: (1) Performing a basic search; (2) Limiting your search; (3) Refining your search using Limit functions; (4) Refining your search using Combine.

Comment

You can search for authors or subjects using the database by typing keyword(s) in this white rectangular box. When you click on the **Perform Search** button, the computer will then match your keyword(s) to the appropriate subject terms. This so called mapping facility is useful as it provides some support in selecting search terms.

NOTE

Whenever a 'Security' dialogue Box appears, simply click on the command Continue

Comment

A list of **subject headings** similar to that shown on the right should appear on your screen.

Notice that *community care* is not a subject heading. (You may need to scroll down (↓) to see the bottom of the list.) This is because CINAHL is an American database.

Starting CINAHL

① Log on to Windows and start your browser.

② Log on to BIOMED: type http://biomed.niss.ac.uk

③ Point and click on CINAHL. *The screen below will be displayed.*

Performing a basic search

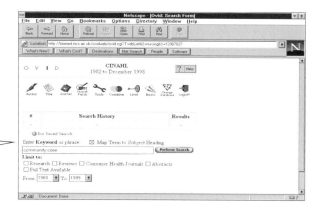

① Point and click on the white rectangular **Search** box. *A flashing cursor should appear inside that box.*

② For this activity, type the keyword(s) **community care** (as shown in the screenshot above) then . . .

③ Point and click on the **Perform Search** button or simply press the RETURN key on the keyboard.

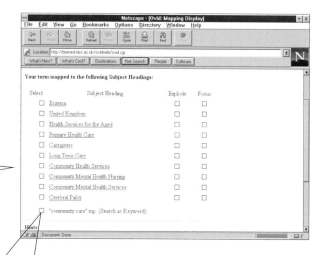

④ Point to the **community care** box and click once. *A cross should appear in the white square box.*

⑤ Point and click on the **Continue** button. You may need to scroll up (↑) to see it. *A screen like the one below should appear.*

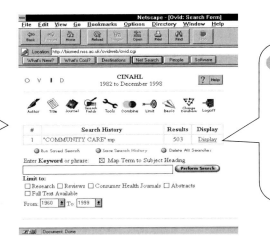

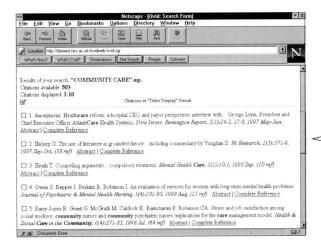

⑦ Point and click on the command **Complete Reference** (The one next to the record no.1).*You should see the screen below appear.*

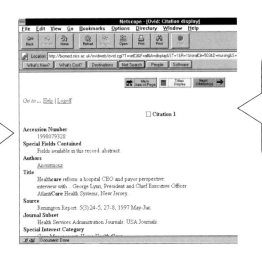

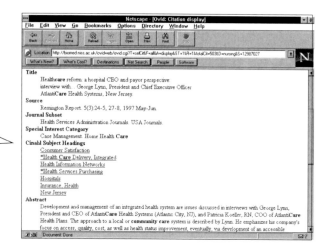

Comment

As you can see some of the subject headings have an asterisk (*) in front of the word(s). These words are what are called the *focus* of the article; ie, they tell you what are the most important topics in the article.

Finally you have an abstract for citation number 1.

9 To see the abstract for the next citation you simply click on the button marked **Next** located at the bottom of the page. Try it now, if you want.

....

THIS BRINGS US TO THE END OF PART ONE

The above steps have shown you how to carry out a basic search on CINAHL and browse through the generated list. As CINAHL is an American database, many of the references may not be appropriate or easily accessible. Also, you may not always wish to browse through 503 records (sometimes hundreds more) to find what you want, as this will be time consuming.

Fortunately there are ways of reducing your search display to a more manageable number. In *Part Two*, we will refine the search we did in Part One by using limit factors provided by the CINAHL database. As you shall see, the **Limit** function allows you to limit your search by a number of criteria.

....

Limiting your search

1 (If you have not already done so), click on the button labelled **Main Search Page**. *Your screen should look like the one shown below.*

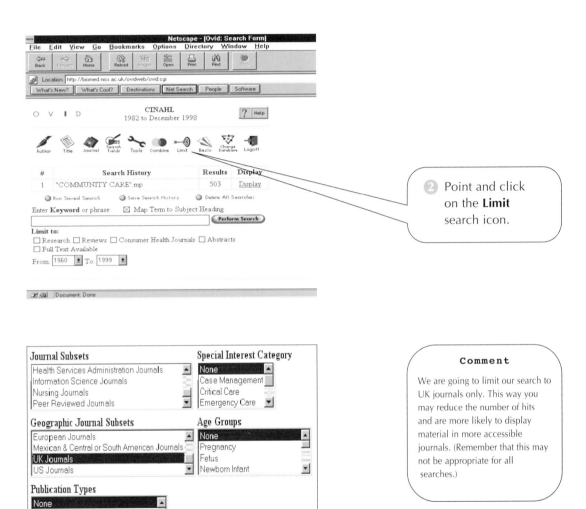

2 Point and click on the **Limit** search icon.

Comment

We are going to limit our search to UK journals only. This way you may reduce the number of hits and are more likely to display material in more accessible journals. (Remember that this may not be appropriate for all searches.)

3 Scroll up (↑) or down(↓) as necessary until you see the display in the screenshot above.

4 Scroll the **Geographic Journal Subsets** window until you see **UK journals**, then click the phrase to highlight it as shown in the screenshot.

5 Click on the **Limit Search** button again. *The search screen below should appear displaying two searches. The second search is UK only. (You may need to scroll up or down to see it.)*

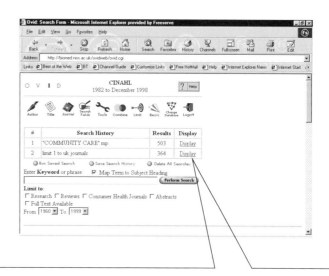

To view your hit point click on this **Display** command and you should see a list showing the first 10 references. To view any of them repeat Steps 7–9 as shown in Part One.

THIS BRINGS US TO THE END OF PART TWO

In Part Three we will carry a more advanced search. But, before moving to the next part we need to reset the system. The easiest way is to click on the **HOME** button on your Browser's toolbar.

Do this now, then go to Part Three.

Refining your search

PART THREE

1. Log on the BIOMED, then point and click on CINAHL.

2. In the **Search** box, type the keyword(s) **mental disorders** and then click on the **Perform Search** button. *A Mapping Display screen as shown in the screenshot below should apprear.*

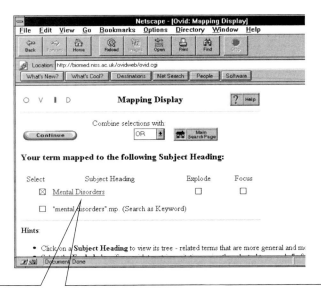

3. Click on the keyphrase **Mental Disorders**. *A **Tree Display** screen like the one below should appear.*

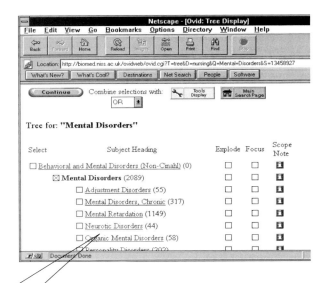

> **Comment**
>
> Notice how the database has provided you with a list of narrower headings associated with **Mental Disorder**.

4. Click on the keyphrase Neurotic Disorders. *Another Tree Display screen as shown below should appear.*

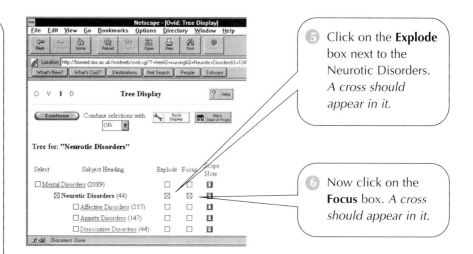

⑤ Click on the **Explode** box next to the Neurotic Disorders. *A cross should appear in it.*

⑥ Now click on the **Focus** box. *A cross should appear in it.*

⑦ Click on the **Continue** button. *A list of Subheadings as shown in the screen below should appear.*

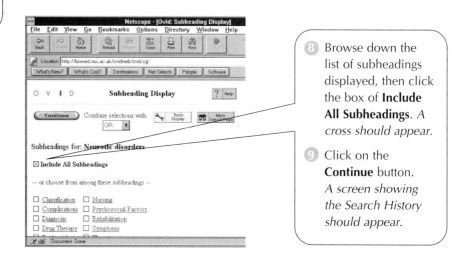

⑧ Browse down the list of subheadings displayed, then click the box of **Include All Subheadings**. *A cross should appear.*

⑨ Click on the **Continue** button. *A screen showing the Search History should appear.*

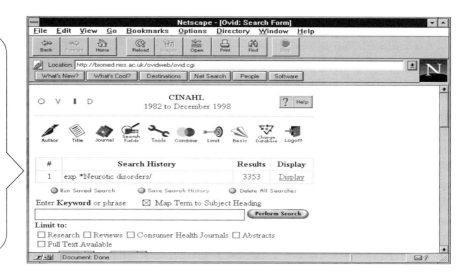

Limit your search to UK Journals only

Do this now by following Steps 1–5 in Part Two. *When you've completed the task, your* **Search History** *list should look something like this:*

#	SEARCH HISTORY	RESULTS	DISPLAY
1	exp *Neurotic disorders/	3353	Display
2	limit 1 to uk journals	524	Display

Limit your search to UK Journals and to Adult 19–44 years

Do this now by following Steps 1–5 in Part Two. *When you've completed the task, your* **Search History** *list should now look something like this:*

#	SEARCH HISTORY	RESULTS	DISPLAY
1	exp *Neurotic disorders/	3353	Display
2	limit 1 to uk journals	524	Display
3	limit 2 to (uk journals and adult <19 to 44 years>)	119	Display

....

THIS BRINGS US TO THE END OF PART THREE

We have looked at how we can limit factors to refine search results. In *Part Four* we will explore another alternative to the **Limit** option, called Combine search.

To use the **Combine** option we need to preserve our current search and carry out a new search.

Off we go.

....

PART FOUR   *Combine search terms*

1 Use the steps 1 to 5 under the heading "*Perform a basic search*" listed in Part One and carry out the search using the keyphrase **community care**. *When you have reached Step 5, your Search History should display four items as shown in the screenshot below.*

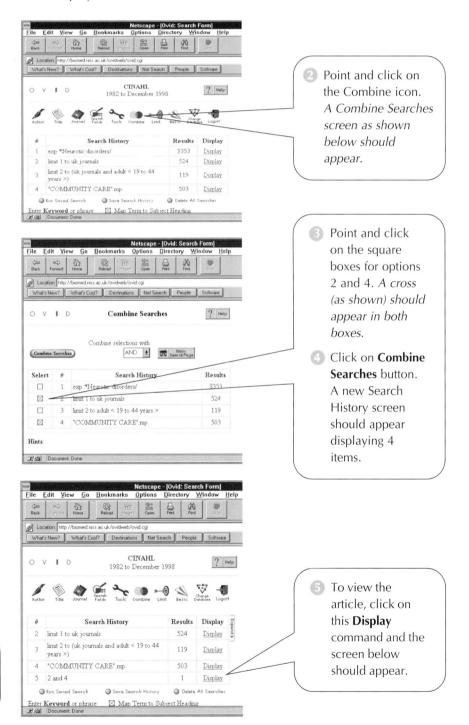

2 Point and click on the Combine icon. *A Combine Searches screen as shown below should appear.*

3 Point and click on the square boxes for options 2 and 4. *A cross (as shown) should appear in both boxes.*

4 Click on **Combine Searches** button. A new Search History screen should appear displaying 4 items.

5 To view the article, click on this **Display** command and the screen below should appear.

Comment

The Combine search option has enabled us to reduce the 1027 (ie, 524+503) articles to 1 article.

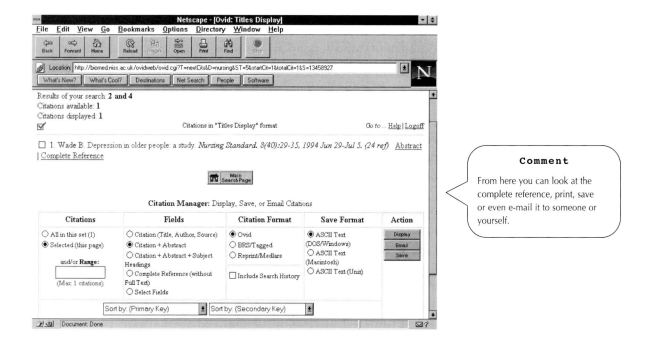

Comment

From here you can look at the complete reference, print, save or even e-mail it to someone or yourself.

4.4 printing your finds

Once you have located the material you want, you can print the entire document or selected pages.

TO PRINT	DO THIS
Entire document	Make sure the printer is Online (ie ready for printing).
	Point and click on the **Print** icon located on your browser's toolbar. If you are printing in a computer lab, your request will be placed in a queue until your turn comes.
Selected pages	Click on the command **File** on the menubar.
	Select the **print** command on the dropdown menu.
	Type the pages you want printed.
	Click on the command **OK**.

summary and conclusion

There are different tools for searching health, medical and general web sites. Some search engines provide better searches in different areas of topics. Try to experiment with them all but remember that some do get busy in the daytime. Remember that Information Gateways can be a very useful starting point when surfing, and that Boolean Operators do provide a way for limiting and broadening the limits of your search.

"Even the many nurses who do not at the moment have ready access to the technology can hardly fail to be aware of the existence of the Internet, and the communication possibilities that exist through e-mail . . ."*Murray (1998)*[10]

Lecturer
School of Health and Social Welfare
The Open University, Milton Keynes.

"Approximately 400 million email messages are sent and received a day over the Internet." *Internet Society*

....

Electronic mail or **e-mail**, is essentially a text system that allows messages to be passed from one user to reach another user who is connected to the Internet or a computer network.

Electronic mail or **e-mail** is one of the most popular, hence most used services on the Internet. As a student of healthcare following a course in a college of higher education or university, after you have registered with your institution's computing services to use their network(s) you will automatically receive an e-mail account. This will not only enable you to send and receive text messages to and from *almost* anyone in the world who has an e-mail account, but you will also be able to send drawings, software, letters prepared using a wordprocessor, documents or reports compiled from a spreadsheet program and so on. They will (nearly always) reach their destination within minutes of being sent. Once you have started to use e-mail, you may find that it becomes your preferred method of communication. Health professionals, too, are beginning to recognise the advantages electronic mail has over other forms of sending or receiving written messages. As Information Systems become more evident in hospital trusts, e-mail will become an integral part of it. The knowledge and skills needed to use this electronic system efficiently are not difficult to learn. Many of your fellow students have already mastered the basics. As long as you are prepared to invest some time and effort, you too can enjoy the benefits of this new technology. This Unit explains the principles of e-mail, discusses issues associated with this system and looks into how to operate Simeon mail – one of the e-mail programs you are most likely to encounter in educational establishments.

checklist

Below is a checklist of what you can expect to find out in this unit. Read through the statements then tick (✓) the items about which you would like to know more.

I would like to find out more about

Please turn over the page and read through the topics you have ticked

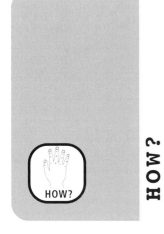

Access code is a unique combination of characters, usually letters or numbers, used in communications as identification for gaining access to a computer. The access code is generally referred to as *Username* or user ID and *password*.

E-mail enables you to send and receive messages without the need for either party to put pen to paper. The message can be as long as you want. This relatively new concept in human communication is, in effect, an electronic post office. However, unlike ordinary mail, the address is not a fixed location like a house, but an individual. Hence the individual can access his/her mailbox from any suitable computer terminal anywhere in the world. Like many other users, e-mail is probably going to be the first Internet application you will come into contact with, and may turn out to be the most important for you. Also if you are worried about e-mail messages that arrive while you are *off-line* (ie, when you are not connected to your service provider's computer), then relax. E-mail will wait for you for a long time.

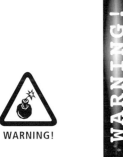

HOW?

How does e-mail work?

When you address an e-mail message to someone or vice versa, the message is stored in a central computer in the recipient's electronic mailbox until (s)he checks whether any messages have been received. At that moment the recipient can inspect it, print it out or reply to it. Messages can be left in someone's e-mail box at any time of night or day and will stay there until collected. (Most mail servers only delete messages that remain uncollected when several months have passed by.) Since the central computer stores thousands of electronic mail boxes including your own, this system makes it possible for you to receive and send mail any where in the world using a unique <u>access code</u>. This <u>access code</u> ensures that users only get the messages intended for them.

As can be expected even with a good system there is a down side. E-mail is no exception. For example:

Downsides of e-mail

▌ it is against the law to send correspondence such as invoices and writs;

▌ if the line being used is too noisy, e-mail messages can be corrupted;

▌ the facility to respond immediately can encourage hasty, thoughtless replies;

▌ a whiz-kid can break into an e-mail box, though this can be minimised by frequent changing of passwords;

▌ when using the Reply option to respond to an e-mail message, a copy may thoughtlessly go to other people.

WARNING!

5.1.1 e-mail programs

To use e-mail, you need an e-mail program. As you can expect, many different programs exist. However, all of them let you do the following:

- Read your incoming mail;
- Send new mail;
- Reply to messages you receive;
- Forward e-mail messages to other people;
- Save messages for later;
- Print e-mail messages.

5.1.2 e-mail headers

Although different e-mail programs look a little different, the important **headers** are the same. Here is a guide to what these lines mean:

table 5.1 **The important e-mail headers**

HEADER	DESCRIPTION
To:	Here you enter the e-mail address of the recipient.
CC:	If you want others to receive a copy of your e-mail, then type their e-mail addresses in this field.
BCC:	If you want to send the same message to someone else or several other people and you do not want the recipient to know who else is getting a copy, place their addresses in this field instead of the CC: field.
From:	Usually your e-mail software will automatically enter your e-mail address in this field. This tells the recipient who to reply to.
Reply To:	Enter the e-mail address you want replies to be sent to (if different than the From: field).
Subject:	Here you can give your e-mail message a short descriptive label. Although you can leave this field blank, it *not* advisable to do so. The label you enter will help the recipient to easily identify the message when (s)he looks for this message again a few months later.
Attachment:	Lists the name of any computer files you want to send to the recipient along with the message.
Date:	Time and date message sent is provided automatically by the software.

Headers are the lines of text that appear at the beginning of every Internet mail message.

NOTE

Many other optional header lines exist, but none of them is of great importance.

To send e-mail to someone, you need his or her address and to receive e-mail you need to have an address. The address lets the computer know how to get the e-mail to the right person. Each e-mail address follows an established format and consists of the following basic parts:

- Mailbox name, which is usually the username of your account;
- @ (the 'at' symbol) separates the username from the location of the server computer.
- Host name or Domain name, which is the address of the Internet Service Provider.

For example, **s.s.chellen@canterbury.ac.uk** is a typical address, where **s.s.chellen** is my mailbox name and **canterbury.ac.uk** is the host name. My mailbox name and the host name are linked by an @ symbol. Hosts are computers that are directly attached to the Internet. Host names have several parts strung together with periods. Fig. 5.1 shows what each part of an e-mail address means.

fig. 5.1 **The anatomy of an e-mail address**

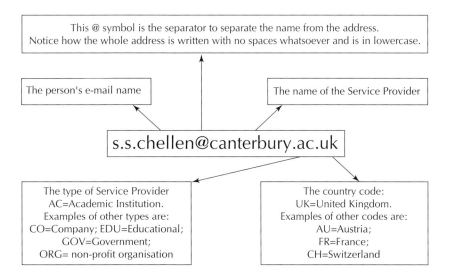

This @ symbol is the separator to separate the name from the address.
Notice how the whole address is written with no spaces whatsoever and is in lowercase.

The person's e-mail name

The name of the Service Provider

s.s.chellen@canterbury.ac.uk

The type of Service Provider
AC=Academic Institution.
Examples of other types are:
CO=Company; EDU=Educational;
GOV=Government;
ORG= non-profit organisation

The country code:
UK=United Kingdom.
Examples of other codes are:
AU=Austria;
FR=France;
CH=Switzerland

Reading e-mail addresses

You may need to verbalise your e-mail address to someone. To avoid sounding like a novice, replace the fullstops in the address with the word 'dot' and the @ sign with the word 'at'.

Thus, my e-mail address would be pronounced 's *dot* s *dot* chellen at canterbury *dot* ac *dot* uk'.

Typing e-mail addresses

Be careful when typing an e-mail address. One typographic mistake will cause the message to come bouncing back to you, never reaching its destination. Ensure that the entire address is written with no spaces.

Finding e-mail addresses

By far the most effective way of finding out the e-mail address of a person or organisation is to ask them. Where this is not possible, it can be quite a problem because as yet there is no complete "Phone Directory" of people's e-mail addresses. Levine et al. (1997)[11] suggest the following strategies:

> When you receive an e-mail message from someone, look at the 'From' field, and you should find the address of message author. Copy it down in your e-mail address book.

> Look at the person's business card or stationery, it may list an e-mail address.

> Try using some of the search engines like Yahoo, AltaVista, DejaNews, and InfoSeek offered on the World Wide Web. You can search on the name of the person or company whose e-mail address you want to find.

Also, all Internet sites that receive e-mail have a person who has the responsibility for sorting out problems with mail. They set up a special e-mail address for this purpose, called "postmaster". So if you have a friend you want to e-mail and you know (s)he has an account with a particular service — say "Demon Internet" — then sending an e-mail to "postmaster@demon.co.uk" can help you to find her/his e-mail address.

HOW?

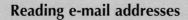

WARNING!

Always remember that all systems managers have access to user files on their systems, making it possible for them to read other people's e-mail. Whether or not they have the time or inclination to do so is anybody's guess. Most system managers probably would not bother, but it is always possible that some can't help being curious. Also, some institutions may have a monitoring policy. The FBI, too, may set up "monitoring" sites along the Internet route.

5.3 using e-mail on a college network

Once you have received your e-mail account from your educational institution, you are ready to start e-mailing any one in the college or anywhere in the world, provided they have an e-mail account.

In this book I will direct you to a website where you will find instructions for using Simeon Mail. You should find that once you have learnt how to use this particular mail program, you should have no difficulty applying the principles covered in this book to other e-mail programs. If you have a different e-mail program at your institution (or at home), your own college website or your service provider may have an online tutorial giving you instructions how to use it.

5.3.1 the mechanics of e-mail

Most e-mail programs allow you to do the following:

Send mail – The message is sent to its destination in Cyberspace.

Receive mail – You can receive mail addressed to your e-mail account.

Reply – You can reply to e-mail you've received.

Forward – You can send a received e-mail message to another person.

Save – You can save e-mail you've received.

Print – You can print e-mail you've received.

Address book – You can store e-mail addresses.

When you send mail, you need to address it to another e-mail user (by typing the person's e-mail name and address). Make sure you have copied down the e-mail address correctly. Here's an example of an e-mail message from me to a colleague using Outlook Express (which is another e-mail program from Microsoft).

fig. 5.2 **A compose-message window**

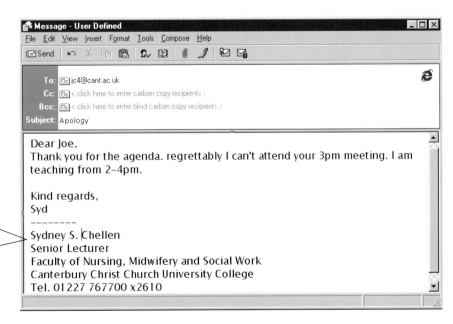

Notice the details in signature at the end of the message? They are usually entered automatically by the e-mail program (read Section 5.7.1, p. 117).

Later on you will have an opportunity to create your signature. First, let's clarify a few things.

5.3.2 undelivered e-mail

When an e-mail message has not been delivered, it is 'bounced' back to you, sometimes immediately and other times after a few days. Your bounced message will be in your **Inbox**, along with an automatically generated explanation of what went wrong. If it bounces immediately, this usually means that the address you have typed doesn't exist, or you made a mistake. Occasionally, there may be a problem in delivering the message at the other end. If this is the reason, then try sending the message again. If the problem persists, address a message to the postmaster asking if there's a problem with e-mail delivery and quoting the e-mail address you were trying to send to. For example, if you were trying to send an e-mail to me, say something like this:

Inbox is a term used to describe the box that stores all your incoming mail until it is read.

I was trying to send an e-mail to:
s.s.chellen@cant.ac.uk
and it bounced.

You can address a message to the postmaster like so:

In the **To:** field, type: ***postmaster@cant.ac.uk***
In the **Text area**, you state that your e-mail to ***s.s.chellen@cant.ac.uk*** has bounced and you would like to know why.

5.3.3 replying to e-mail messages

If you have received an e-mail, you can send a reply without having to type the sender's e-mail address and text. For example, let's assume you have received an e-mail and you have opened it into your **Viewer** window, as shown in the screenshot below.

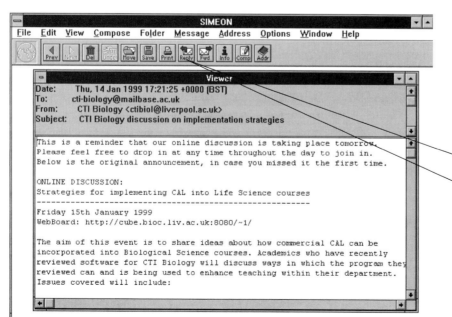

Once you have read the message, to reply to it you just point and click on the **Reply** icon on Simeon's toolbar.

A Reply window, as shown in the next screenshot, will open up.

108

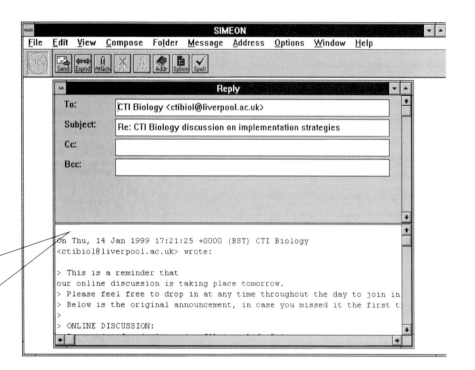

Simeon will automatically fill in the address and subject for you. It will also copy the original message into your text area.

A cursor should be flashing where the arrow is pointing. If this not the case, place your pointer there and click the left mouse button.

As you start typing your reply it will push down the original text. When you are ready click on the **Send** button. Providing there are no errors, after the message has been posted the **Reply** window should close down.

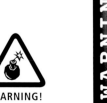

Using Reply to answer e-mail messages

Be very careful to check all the return addresses Simeon fills in for you — if the mail was addressed to more than one person, you'll be replying to all of them, which may not be what you want. So trim out the addresses you do not want. You can also trim the quoted text as much as you possibly can. It is considered very bad manners to quote someone's entire mail message just to add a one-line reply.

Forwarding e-mail and the law

Forwarding e-mail you have received in your Inbox is so easy to do and quite a common practice, but beware as you might be infringing someone's copyright. Steve Gilligan, a learning technology advisor from TLTSN centre at the University of Bangor and a specialist in copyright on the Internet, points out during a seminar at the University of Kent that although 'e-mail is something we take for granted these days, all e-mail received from others is subject to copyright protection ie, the person who creates an e-mail holds the copyright of that composition'. He added 'if you intend to distribute (ie, forward) e-mail that you have received, then you should have the permission of that person before doing so'.

Gilligan suggested further that 'under normal conditions an e-mail message will contain information about the origin of the e-mail. This is normally adequate for the purposes of attributing a work to a person. Editing of such e-mail which may mislead people into thinking that, for example, an original idea expressed in someone else's e-mail is in fact coming from you, is an infringement of their copyright'. He added that 'e-mail is subject to the laws of libel and defamation' and concluded that 'e-mail has been successfully used in recent libel cases'. So, be careful what you write and to whom.

If you are ready and have Simeon Mail program installed on your WINDOWS NT workstation or your own computer, carry out the tasks listed in Activity 5.1.

▶ Get on the Net. Type the URL below in your **Address/Location** box of your browser, then press the ENTER key. After a few seconds an online tutorial should appear. It contains instructions on how to: ***activate Simeon, read, send, reply to***, and ***forward*** e-mail-messages. Also how to ***print, save*** and ***quit*** Simeon. Use the on-screen instructions and obtain a print out of the tutorial **SimPart1.htm.**

> http://www.cant.ac.uk/title/Simeon/Part1/SimPart1.htm

▶ Using the appropriate instructions in the print out, send a short e-mail message to a friend in your college or elsewhere, then close down Simeon. At a later time/date re-start Simeon and if you have received a response, read it, get a print out of the message and then make a reply.

When you have completed the activity return to this page and read on

5.3.4 attaching files

Until recently all e-mail messages could only consist of ASCII text – ie, the characters you see on your keyboard, with no formatting features like bold, italics, underline, and no drawing or fancy layout. This meant that, if you wanted to design a questionnaire to collect health data for a particular assignment, you would not have been able to make use of those formatting features mentioned above to enhance presentation. But, with Simeon Mail (and most other modern e-mail programs) you can now "attach" one or more files to an e-mail message. The attachment can be a word processing file, a chart from a spreadsheet, an image etc. This is a very powerful facility that you can exploit to your advantage. Now you can use a wordprocessor to prepare your questionnaire. You can lay it out the way you would like it to look, using any formatting features you want. When you are satisfied with your design, you can save it to disk as you would do with any document file. You can also prepare a covering letter to accompany the questionnaire.

When you are ready to send out your questionnaire, you simply attach it to a short e-mail message. In it you should advise your recipients that when they have completed the questionnaire, they should use the '**Forward**' function to return the e-mail back to you.

While Simeon is sending your e-mail, it will automatically encode the attached file(s), so that it can be sent successfully. When Simeon receives a message with an attachment, it decodes the file, and places it on your hard disk. Activity 5.2 will help you send an e-mail with attachment.

> **NOTE**
>
> When preparing a covering letter to accompany your attached file(s), it is useful to inform your recipient(s) of the kind of document you are attaching. For example, stating that it is a document prepared using Word 6.0. This way if your recipients have a problem retrieving the attachment the information given might explain why.

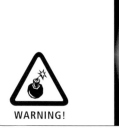

'Attachment' problems

In some cases attaching files to e-mail can be tricky, especially when your recipient's e-mail program cannot handle them, usually because their program is using a different conversion system. If you know that your software and that of your recipient both use the same system, attaching files is very simple, and works well.

activity 5.2 ATTACHING FILES TO AN E-MAIL MESSAGE

1. Using your word processor, construct a one-page questionnaire to collect data about the smoking habits of students attending your course, and save it to your hard disk in a directory where you will be able to find it or on a floppy disk.

2. Pay a visit to this website: http://www.cant.ac.uk/title/Simeon/Part2/ SimPart2.htm It contains, amongst other things, instructions on how to attach a file to an e-mail message. Get a printout of the tutorial: **SimPart2.htm**

3. Now, randomly select the e-mail addresses of the six students on your course, who will receive your questionnaire.

4. Using the instructions in **SimPart2.htm**, e-mail the questionnaire to the chosen students as an attachment. Ask them to complete and forward it back to you.

When you have completed the activity return to this page and read on

5.3.5 deleting or moving incoming mail

Once you have read your e-mail from your Inbox, it is good practice to either delete it from your provider's mail server or move it to a folder. This is because your provider won't give you unlimited space for e-mail on the server. When your Inbox is full, incoming mail will just bounce back to the sender. You may receive a reminder from the System Manager requesting that you clean your Inbox. Failure to respond to such a request may result in your Inbox being cleaned for you. The process of deleting or moving e-mail is quite simple. Before you can move an e-mail message, you must have a folder ready to move the e-mail into. This too is quite easy to create, as you will find out by carrying out the tasks in Activity 5.3.

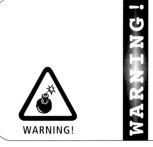
Be extra careful when deleting messages, because once you have deleted an e-mail message you may not be able to get it back.

5.3.6 creating folders

Most e-mail programs (including Simeon Mail) enable you to save messages that are similar or deal with the same subject in folders. After you save a message to a folder, you can later on call that folder up again and open all the messages in it. Organising messages in this way can save you valuable time when searching for old messages. In the screenshot below you can see there is a *tree* with a long list of various folders that I have created for my own use.

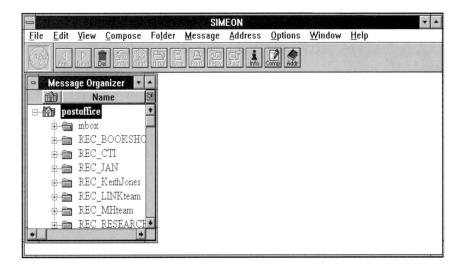

The steps for creating a folder to add to the tree are quite simple. In the next activity you will have an opportunity to create a folder.

activity 5.3

Using the instructions in the online tutorial worksheets: **SimPart1** and **SimPart2**, practise the following:

1. Forwarding e-mail messages;
2. Saving an e-mail message to a file;
3. Printing an e-mail message;
4. Deleting and Undeleting e-mail messages;
5. Creating a new folder;
6. Transferring messages to other folders.

When you have completed the activity return to this page and read on

5.4 what you need to use e-mail at home

If you would like to send and receive e-mail from the comfort of your home, then you will need a few bits and pieces. You may have a few of them already. The activity below will help you identify your current situation.

activity 5.4 WHAT DO YOU NEED?

Here is a list of what you will need to be able to send and receive e-mail from the comfort of your home. Use this checklist to tick (✓) your requirements:

- a computer;
- a *modem* to use with your computer;
- a telephone line to connect your modem;
- communication *software*;
- membership of a *service provider* to get on the Internet;
- an electronic name and address. (This will be issued to you by the service provider.);
- the electronic name and address of the person you are attempting to communicate with.

For more information on the items listed above, please refer to Unit 2, Section 2.3.

There are some simple unwritten rules that you are expected to follow when posting electronic mail messages. These are known widely as netiquette. These rules are equally applicable to postings on bulletin boards, commercial online services, and mailing lists. Obeying these rules can make e-mail more useful and effective. Rinaldi[12] offers a well-respected guide. Here are a few DOs and DON'Ts:

table 5.2 **E-mail netiquette**

DO'S	DON'TS
keep your messages short – this makes them quicker to read and more likely to get a reply, especially by busy individuals;	send junk mail – it clogs up the system unnecessarily;
use white space in the message rather than lumping all the text together, and do number your topics or create new paragraphs. These make reading easier.	use too many words in CAPITAL LETTERS. They are difficult to read and in e-mail this is perceived as yelling and can provoke an angry response;
be kind to your reader. Punctuate your message properly. Messages that do not use capitals to begin sentences and proper nouns are hard to read.	use words that denigrate someone – libelling someone in an e-mail is an offence;
include a snippet of the e-mail you are replying to – it puts your message in context;	reply in heated verbal terms. In e-mail lingo, this is referred to as "flaming".
test your recipients' capability of reading an e-mail attachment before sending one. There is no point in sending an attachment to someone if (s)he cannot access it.	forward someone's private e-mail without his or her permission.
keep *signatures* short and relevant (see Section 5.7.1).	use culturally specific language as a general rule. UK colloquialisms or metaphors may not be understood abroad.
	assume that your e-mail is confidential; others may be able to read or access your mail. Therefore, refrain from sending or keeping anything that you would mind seeing on the evening news.

WARNING!

Flaming health professionals

A *"flame"* is an inflammatory criticism directed at another e-mail user. This situation can easily occur with messages sent to newsgroups. A "flame war" can quickly erupt when other users flame those doing the criticising. Doctors, nurses and other health professionals are sometimes targets for vicious attacks on their personal character and professional reputation by people who are hostile for no apparent reason.

How to cope with e-mail overload

When people find themselves overloaded with e-mail messages, this inevitably leads them to avoid reading their e-mail. This is usually not a useful solution for anyone to adopt as it reduces the benefits of an e-mail system. Here are some strategies that you could use to reduce the problem of overload:

▶ <u>Be Selective</u> (a) When sending e-mail to a number of recipients, decide whether what you are writing is pertinent to all of them. If not, then do not include them on the list of recipients. (b) When you are replying to an e-mail message that has been sent to multiple recipients, the system will usually ask you if you want your reply to go to "all" recipients. You should only select "yes" if your response is pertinent to all of them.

▶ <u>Good Housekeeping</u> Delete unwanted e-mail and sort and save useful ones in folders. You could create intray folders to help you prioritise your reading and reply of e-mail — for example *Very urgent, Moderate, not urgent.*

▶ <u>Keep to a single idea</u> When writing your e-mail, each message should deal with one topic only. This will reduce the length of the message and encourage your reader to read the message.

▶ <u>Adopt a business style</u> Keep your message business-like. The formality, topics, language, and routing of your e-mail should follow business rules.

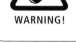

Composing your e-mail while being online

When using the network at your college/university, you will normally be composing your e-mail while being online. This is costing your institution more in phone bills and you may not be able to do anything about that. However, when using your own system at home, remember that you only need to be connected when you are fetching or sending mail. So, check the program you are using and see if it is possible to compose your e-mail message off-line.

5.6 using keyboard characters to convey feelings

A bit of humour when sending e-mail can be a nice touch, but making funny remarks on e-mail can quite easily be taken as deep and deadly insults which could result in a 'flaming' war online.

In face to face conversations, or even on the phone, there are all sorts of clues that indicate the real meaning behind words which help one to determine whether what is being said should be taken affectionately or angrily. On e-mail, this can be difficult but not impossible. Emotions, otherwise known as 'smileys', are little expressive faces that can be made from standard keyboard characters to convey feelings or to prevent a comment being misunderstood in e-mail messages, newsgroups postings and text-chat. As an example, you may put <s> (for smiling) or <g> (for grinning) at the end of a sentence to say to the reader: 'I am joking'. Here are some recognised smileys:

table 5.3   **Some keyboard characters conveying emotion**

SYMBOL	MEANING
:-)	Indicates a smile or a humorous remark.
;-)	Signifies a wink, a joke, or a sarcastic comment.
:-(	Indicates a frown or depressing remark.
%-)	Expresses confusion.
:-> or >:-)	Signifies a devilish grin.
:-||	Indicates you are angry.
:-|	Indicates you are not amused.
:-&	Indicates you are tongue-tied.

If you can't make any sense of the above symbols, try turning this page sideways.

By the way, also in common usage are acronyms which came about as a result of Internet users having to compose their e-mail while online and clocking up charges. Although messages can now be composed offline, the use of acronyms has become a part of accepted e-mail style, and you will find them if you get involved with Chat. You can turn just about any phrase into so-called acronyms. Here is a little bundle of them:

table 5.4   **Some acronyms used in e-mail**

SYMBOL	MEANING
AFAIK	As far as I know
BCNU	Be seeing you
BTW	By the way
FAQ	Frequent asked question(s)
FWIW	For what it's worth
FYI	For your information
IMO	In my opinion
IOW	In other words
OAO	Over and out
OTOH	On the other hand
OTT	Over the top
TNX	Thanks

NOTE

When sending e-mail messages, if the e-mail program you are using does not allow the use of bold, italic or underline to emphasise particular words or phrases. You can do the following:
To emphasise text you can surround the word or phrase with asterisks or underline like so: (*bold*), (_underscore_).

WARNING!

Don't confuse your reader

However interesting, amusing or even useful acronyms and smileys might be, they unfortunately breed a very confusing style of communication. They have been included in this book simply to increase your awareness of their existence. If you must use them, then do so with great caution, for just because you know that *IMHO* stands for '*In my humble opinion*', it doesn't mean that anyone else does.

NOTE

When trying a new option, you can check it out by sending a test-message to yourself.

Modern e-mail programs tend to offer more than the basic requirements of composing, sending, receiving and reading. Spending a little time finding what else your e-mail program can do is always time well spent. Here are two options than you ought to investigate when you have a moment or two.

5.7.1 signatures

You can finish off your e-mail messages by adding details about yourself which are not provided by the mail headers. For example, your name, telephone and fax numbers, the course you are on and a motto. It would be tedious to have to type out all this information every time you compose an e-mail. Signature is an option on one of your program's menus. This option provides a blank space for you to enter whatever text you choose, and this will be automatically added to the end of all the messages you write. Signatures can be fun for a while, but if someone gets a lot of mail messages from you, a signature that takes up a lot of space can soon end up boring. As a rule of thumb, keep your signature as short as possible – in any case it should never be more than 4 lines. The longer your signature, the lower you are held in esteem by many people on the Net.

5.7.2 address books

This is simply a facility, available in most e-mail programs, for you to compile a list of names and e-mail addresses. This way, whenever you need to send some-one an e-mail, instead of having to type his or her e-mail address, you can select it from your address book and it will be inserted in the correct place for you. With programs like Simeon, you can also create multiple address books, or you can group addresses into different categories for speedy access. Being able to group addresses is quite useful, for example, when you need to send the same message to all the members listed in that group, you simply double-click the group name.

activity 5.5   CREATE AN ADDRESS BOOK AND SIGNATURE FILE

Using the printout from the online tutorial: **SimPart2.htm**, do the following:

▶ Create an address book in Simeon;
▶ Create a signature file.

summary and conclusion

E-mail is relatively a new form of communications. It can be less expensive, and often more informative than a telephone conversation. You can send an e-mail all over the world for a very little expense and it will reach its destination in seconds. You can attach spreadsheets, drawings and lots more. Do remember to follow the netiquette and you will find e-mailing a fun way to communicate with other healthcare users.

"Joining a Mailbase discussion list is an invaluable method for keeping up-to-date in your area of interest. The lists can range from broad disciplines such as public health and psychiatric nursing which provide a discussion forum for related issues and highlight new initiatives, developments, conferences etc, to extremely focused lists such as pupil or acupuncture."
Howson (1998).[13]

Information Officer,
ScHARR – University of Sheffield
e-mail: n.j.howson@sheffield.ac.uk

"There are over 25,000 different newsgroups covering every topic you could think of."

Internet Society

The sheer range of opportunities the Internet offers is beyond belief. In the previous unit we discussed e-mail. Besides exchanging e-mail messages with colleagues or other health professionals you can also join **Newsgroups** – more formally known as Usenet discussion groups. You can find newsgroups on any subject. There are an estimated twenty-eight thousand or more newsgroups and hundreds of them are groups concerned with health issues. By joining one or more of these discussion groups you will be able to share your views with other healthcare students or health professionals. Each newsgroup provides a forum for discussion of issues related to a specialist subject. As a participant you will be able to engage around the clock in group discussions, trade information and ideas with other healthcare colleagues on the far side of the world. This is a great and fun way to test your thoughts on particular health issues.

Another useful and interesting way for people of shared interests to send e-mail messages to each other, is via **Mailing Lists**. Mailing lists differ from newsgroups in that a separate copy of the mailing list message is e-mailed to each recipient on the list. By and large mailing lists are more intimate than newsgroups, more specific, usually less riotous and you can participate regardless of what kind of service provider you have, just as long as you can send and receive e-mail.

In this unit we will uncover some interesting health newsgroups and mailing lists, look at the software you need to access them (both at home or at your institution) and discuss relevant issues.

A Newsgroup is a collection of messages posted by individuals to a news server. A News server is a computer (or program) dedicated to transferring the contents of newsgroups around the Net, and to and from your computer. This may be referred to as an NNTP server. These computers are maintained by companies, organisations and individuals, and can host thousands of newsgroups.

Mailing List This term has two meanings: (a) a list of e-mail addresses to which you can send the same message without making endless copies of it, all with different addresses inserted; and (b) a discussion group similar to newsgroups, but all the messages sent to the group are forwarded to its members by e-mail.

TECHNO TALK

checklist

Below is a checklist of what you can expect to find out in this unit. Read through the statements then tick (✓) the items about which you would like to know more.

I would like to find out more about:

Please turn over the page and read through the topics you have ticked

Posting –
When you
send an e-mail
message, the word
'sending' is quite good enough.
When you send a message to a
newsgroup, it isn't. Instead, for
no adequately explained reason,
the word 'posting' is used, and
the word 'article' is used to
describe the message itself.

Usenet news system is a
worldwide bulletin board system
that allows you to take part in
discussions on a wide range of
topics and is the main public
discussion space on the Net.

Oddly enough Newsgroups have very little to do with "news", as in current events etc. Newsgroups can be described as a public discussion space on the Net (Holyer, 1996).[3] In Unit 5 we looked at e-mail. While e-mail is generally one-to-one communication, newsgroups are one-to-many communication. Discussions take place using e-mail messages (referred to as **postings** or **articles**). Instead of addressing articles to an individual's e-mail address they're addressed to a particular group. Anyone choosing to access this group can read the messages, post replies, initiate new topics of conversation, or even ask questions relating to the subject covered by the group. Some newsgroups are monitored, but most are not. There are no newsgroup membership lists or joining fees.

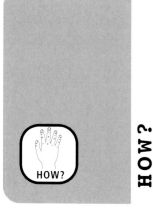

How do newsgroups work?

Your College or Internet Service Provider (ISP) must have a *news server* or a link to one. The news server holds articles from thousands of newsgroups that form part of the Usenet news system. Once you have set up an account with the news server, you can post messages to a particular group. These messages go to the access provider's server, and are then passed from one server to another (a message takes about a day to go around the world). The messages can then be read by anyone who "belongs" to that group, and readers can post replies in the same way as they would compose and send e-mail messages. Articles that you post are added to the server's listings almost immediately and are gradually distributed to other news servers around the world.

6.1.1 newsgroup names

Usenet newsgroups are arranged in hierarchies. Here is an example: **comp.sys.ibm.pc**. As you can see, the names begin with words separated by dots. Reading the names from left to right, they begin with a top-level category name and gradually become more specific. In the example above, the newsgroup is part of the *comp* hierarchy, which is generally to do with computers. The *sys* identifies it as being concerned with a specific computer system, rather than (says) a programming language; the *ibm* and the *pc* elements identify it as covering PCs and compatibles.

Although at first glance, there is a bewildering number of newsgroups, almost all newsgroups that you will be interested in can be classified under eight headings as outlined in Table 6.1.

table 6.1 **Newsgroups of interest to the health professional**

HIERARCHY	DESCRIPTION
sci	Science-related groups eg, **sci.med.nursing** (a general forum); **sci.med.occupational**; **sci.med.dentistry**; **sci.med.pharmacy**; **sci.med.diseases.mental**
soc	The social groups cover social topics and cultural issues eg, **soc.culture.welsh** A very valuable set of *soc* groups is the **soc.support**. This covers a range of mainly long-term and non-life-threatening illnesses eg, **soc.support.depression.crisis**; **soc.support.depression.family**; **soc.support.pregnancy.loss** These can be a lifeline for sufferers and their relatives.
talk	Debates and discussions about controversial topics eg, **talk.euthanasia** **talk.abortion**
uk	Most of the Usenet is international in scope. In practice this means that it is overwhelmingly dominated by Americans. Reflecting this, every country outside of the USA has its own set of newsgroups. The UK-only groups cover a wide range of subjects. *Useful ones to try are*: **uk.misc** **uk.sci.med.nursing** **uk.people.support.epilepsy** (an Epilepsy general discussion group)
misc	Topics that don't fit anywhere else – eg, items for sale, education, investments and also some with relevance to nursing and healthcare, eg, **misc.health.therapy.occupational** **misc.health.infertility** **misc.handicap** **misc.health.aids**
comp	In these groups you will find all sorts of things which are directly related to computers eg, **comp.sys.ibm.pc.** This is probably the most useful comp group, where you can find advice from all over the world about using and setting up IBM-compatible PCs.
news	Groups that deal with the administration of the Usenet news system. New groups are discussed on **news.config**; New groups are announced on **news.announce**. One news group that you should look at is **news.announce.conferences** which carries a range of conferences.
rec	The recreation groups cover a wide range of entertainment topics. These groups are usually fairly gentle and helpful, and are a good place for a beginner (generally nobody will be rude to you if you say the wrong thing). Several recreation groups carry reviews eg, **rec.arts.books.reviews**. These are well worth following, since the reviews are by normal Internet users (ie, probably with similar taste to you).

In addition to the eight hierarchies outlined in Table 6.1, there are several hierarchies that are widely distributed. Table 6.2 shows three examples:

table 6.2 **Other newsgroups which may cover health topics**

HIERARCHY	DESCRIPTION
alt	This group is not an official part of the Usenet service, but is still available from almost all service providers. This group covers alternative topics, often of a bizarre and controversial nature, eg, **alt.support.spina-bifida** **alt.education.disabled** **alt.nurse** **alt.society.mental-health** **alt.support.diabetes.kids**
bionet	Topics of interest to biologists eg, **bionet.biology.cardiovascular** **bionet.audiology**
k12	Topics of interest to elementary and high school students and teachers
bit	Topics of interest for student nurses and others, eg, **Bit.listserv.snurse-l** **bit.listserv.medforum**

NOTE

Many groups are moderated. There are strict controls on the creation of newsgroups: a long and involved process of proposal, debate and finally an Internet-wide vote is necessary.

However, in the <u>alt</u> hierarchy, almost anyone can set up a group. The sole difference from other hierarchies is that their creators can bypass all the red tape involved in the Usenet process. Much of the pornography is available through alt newsgroups.

6.1.2 reading articles

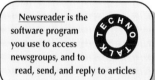

Newsreader is the software program you use to access newsgroups, and to read, send, and reply to articles

In order to read articles you need a program called a **newsreader**. There are a number of newsreader programs available and they basically fall into two types. The first type can be described as *online* newsreader. (If you are planning to use an Internet system at home to read articles, you should avoid this type because to read and post articles you need to be connected, thus clocking up charges.) A better type is the *offline* newsreader.

WARNING!

Beware, since some offline readers automatically *download* all the unread articles in your chosen group so that you can read them and compose replies offline. The downside is that in a popular group you may have to wait for hundreds of articles to download, many of which may not be of interest to you. A really good type of offline reader is the one that just downloads the headers of the articles (ie, the subject line, date, author and size). Based on this information, you can then select the articles you want to read and reconnect to download your selection.

NOTE

In <u>NetScape Navigator 3.0</u> the newsreader is built right in, whereas with <u>NetScape Communicator 4.0</u> the news program is separated and is called <u>NetScape Collabra</u>.

So, if you have your own Internet system at home and you need a good *offline newsreader*, try *Free Agent*. This is a popular newsreader and, as the name suggests, it is free. However, if you already have *Microsoft Internet Explorer* installed on your machine, you will find that the newsreader program is separated and is called *Outlook Express* (which includes both Mail and News).

For our next activity I will use the newsreader Outlook Express to show you how to use the **Online Help** to get started with newsgroups. If you're using anything else, for example Agent or NetScape, you will have the same online help available. By the way, do take note that to read news (be it at the college or at home), you first need to subscribe to the group or groups that interest you. This does not mean that you have to pay fees, but simply that you need to let your newsreader know which group(s) to download headers from.

USING YOUR HOME OR COLLEGE SYSTEM TO READ ARTICLES   activity **6.1**

It is assumed that you have *Microsoft Outlook Express 5.0 installed* on your college WINDOWS NT workstation or on your home system, and that the program is configured for you to be able to join Newsgroups. If this is not the case, the Helpdesk at your institution or your Service Provider should be able to help you.

1. Carry out the steps listed in **Worksheet 10**. They will help you obtain three printouts as follows: How to: (a) *Subscribe to newsgroups'*, (b) *'Posting messages to newsgroups'* and (c) *'Reply to a newsgroup message'*.

2. When you have obtained all three printouts, use the instructions in the appropriate printout and subscribe to two newsgroups of your choice.

When you have completed the activity return to this page and read on

If you have successfully carried out the above activity, you should bear in mind that the other subscribers have no way of knowing that you are now a subscriber. All you have done is told your browser what to ask for. You are now ready to fetch and read articles but you are advised not to rush into posting anything. Just spend a few weeks or months snooping on the group(s) you have chosen.

6.1.3 keeping the cost down

By now you would have discovered that there is nothing difficult about fetching and reading articles. You can use Outlook Express, NetScape or even Agent to read articles in two ways:

▷ If you are not worried about keeping the phone bill down, you can operate any of the above programs in its online mode. This means that your Newsreader is connected to the News server all the time you are reading articles, and collecting them one at a time.

▷ If you want to keep the phone bill down you can set up your Newsreader to operate offline. This means that your Newsreader will fetch new message headers, collect messages you wish to read, and send any responses you may have set up all in one go. You can then read news offline, while you are not running up the phone bill (reading and replying to articles is the most time-consuming part).

Outlook Express

VERSION 5.0

1 Identify the icon labelled **Outlook Express (OE)** and double-click on it. *A dialog box for you to connect to your service provider may appear. Opt for working offline. The OE window should now be clearly visible.*

2 Point and click on the **Help** command on OE menubar. *A submenu should appear.*

3 Click on the key-phrase **"Contents and Index"**. *A dialog box labelled 'Outlook Express Help' – as shown below – should appear.*

4 Click on the section labelled **'Viewing and Posting to Newsgroups'**. *A picklist of items should appear.*

Comment

From here you can select any item you want to know more about. For example to select *"Subscribe to a newsgroup"*, simply point and click on it once and its content will appear in the window on the right. You can then read it Online and also request a printout of it.

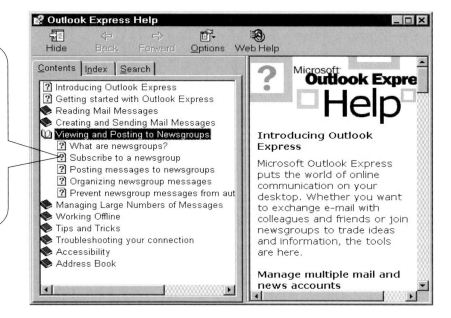

5 Request a printout on the following: **Subscribe to a newsgroup, Posting messages to newsgroups,** and **Reply to a newsgroup message**. To print your selection click on **Options** on the toolbar then select Print.

The strategy then is for you to be more disciplined in reading articles. First you connect to get the headers, and then you connect again to fetch the bodies of any messages you want to read.

6.1.4 old news

Although the headers are displayed, sometimes you may find that some of the articles are no longer available. This is because old articles have to be deleted to make room for new ones. In popular groups, articles may vanish within a matter of days.

> Occasionally you may come across a message that looks like gibberish. It is possible that the message has been encrypted with a program called *ROT13*. This program is used to scramble a message to prevent anyone from accidentally reading it, as it may be nasty. The reader can decide whether or not to read it.

WARNING!

6.1.5 newsgroup netiquette

You can learn a lot by just reading articles. However, you can learn even more by getting involved ie, by contributing constructively to the discussion. However, before posting anything remember that the e-mail etiquette discussed in Unit 5 Section 5.5, applies even more than ever to articles posted to newsgroups. Newsgroups are quite hot on netiquette. Levine et al. (1997)[11] offer the following useful DOs and DONT's. Most of them have been slightly adapted and reproduced in the Warning box on p. 127.

6.1.6 posting your first article

Trying anything for the first time is both exciting and a little bit scary. A completely new news message is called a *posting*. If you reply to someone else's posting, it's called a *follow-up*. You can follow-up to newsgroups, by e-mail to individuals, or both at once.

Here are a few rules that you can follow when you are ready to post your first article. They can make the difference between you enjoying the experience and making you wish you never got involved.

NOTE

Some Newsgroups are moderated, generally by unpaid volunteers, which means instead of articles being posted directly as news, they must be posted to a person or program who only posts the article if (s)he or it feels that it's appropriate to the group.

▶ Pick a newsgroup whose subject is one you know something about.

▶ Learn as much as you can about the group by reading the FAQ. Many groups post FAQ every few weeks. If you can 't see any FAQ, send an e-mail to the group asking if someone could send you one.

▶ Read the original article and other people's replies to make sure that your point has not already been raised.

▶ When replying to an article be certain of your facts (be ready to cite references) and make sure that what you have to say is relevant to the topic being discussed.

▶ Keep your reply short, clear and to the point.

▶ Pay attention to your spelling and grammar.

▶ Avoid 'flaming' others with provocative words. Personal attacks in newsgroups can get so out of hand that the whole group descends into what is known on the Net as 'flame-war'. Don't be the one to start one.

▶ Read your reply over and over before posting it.

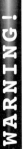

WARNING!

1. Don't post a follow-up to the whole group that is intended solely for the author of the original article. Instead reply via e-mail.

2. Don't post a message saying that another message — for example, a spam ad — is inappropriate. The poster probably knows and doesn't care. Silence is golden.

3. Never criticise someone else's spelling or grammar.

4. If you have to complain about an article, send an e-mail to the post-master at the sender's host.

5. Always make your subject line as meaningful as possible.

6. Be sure that each article is appropriate for the group to which you post it.

7. If you are asking a question, always end your question with a question mark '?'.

8. Don't post a two-line follow-up that quotes an entire 100-line article. Edit out most of the quoted material.

9. Don't cross-post (ie, post the same article to multiple newsgroups) unless there is a really good reason. Be especially careful when replying to multiple cross-posted messages.

10. Watch out for trolls ie, messages calculated to provoke a storm of replies. Remember that not every stupid comment needs a response.

11. Most groups periodically post a list of Frequently Asked Questions (FAQ). Do read FAQ before asking a question as you may find your query has already been answered.

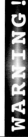

As already mentioned, Usenet Newsgroups are public forum. Everything you say can be read by anyone, anywhere in the world. Moreover, every word you post is carefully indexed and archived. A simple search on your name displays your e-mail address and a list of every message you have ever posted. So, be careful what personal details you include in your message.

POSTING AND FOLLOW-UPS OF ARTICLES TO NEWSGROUPS   activity **6**.2

Newsgroup messages work just like e-mail: the only difference is that the address you use is the name of a newsgroup, not an e-mail address. You post a newsgroup article just as you would send an e-mail message.

Using the instructions in the printouts '*Posting messages to newsgroups*' and '*Reply to a newsgroup message* (which you obtained in Activity 6.1):

1. Compose a one line article and post it to a newsgroup.

2. Select and make a sensible reply to the author of an article.

When you have completed the activity return to this page and read on

Attachments are usually not permitted in newsgroups. The charter for uk.sci.med.nursing definitely doesn't (see www.damien.purplenet.co.uk to read the whole charter).

6.1.7 online help

Both *Outlook Express* and *NetScape* come with excellent online help. While carrying out the activity 6.1, you would have found the option Help on the Menubar. Each time you are not sure how to do something, simply click on Help and select 'Contents and Index'. You'll find lots more information to help you use the many features of your newsreader. Often included are useful tips.

6.1.8 posting header fields

The headers of News postings are very important and can get quite involved. Table 6.3 offers a few suggestions:

table 6.3 **Suggested header fields for News postings**

HEADER FIELDS	COMMENTS
Newsgroups	This contains the newsgroup(s) to which the message will be posted. When putting more than one group in, you should separate the names with commas.
Subject	Whenever you decide to change the subject of a follow-up, it is generally expected that you will include the old subject in brackets. For example a follow-up to a posting called "UK nursing vacancies" could be "Nursing vacancies in Kent (was: UK nursing vacancies)".
e-mail to:	If you put an e-mail address(es) in this field, the message will also be e-mailed to them.
Follow-up to:	If your posting is followed up, this group will be filled in as the defaults group to post to. So, if you are putting a request about vacancies in the UK to a number of groups, but want all follow-ups to go to alt.nurse, put alt.nurse in the Follow-up To field. If you put "poster" in this field, follow-ups will be e-mailed to you (the poster).
Distribution	Use this field to limit how far the posting will be passed on to news servers. For example, if your posting is only relevant to UK, put in the distribution field "uk".
Expires:	To prevent servers deciding on your behalf when your article expires, put a date in this field.

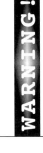

A **thread** is an ongoing topic of conversation in a newsgroup or mailing list. When someone posts a message with a new Subject line they're starting a new thread. Any replies to this message (and replies to replies, and so on) will have the same Subject line and continue the thread.

WARNING!

In a follow-up, check the groups listed very carefully. It's considered bad manners to follow up to inappropriate groups. Also:

When replying to an existing <u>thread</u>, you must not change the subject line at all! If just one character is different, newsreaders will regard it as the start of a new thread and won't group it with the other articles in the thread, so your reply might be overlooked by the very people who would find it most interesting.

6.1.9 asking for help from newsgroups

If you have got a technical problem, one of the Usenet discussion newsgroups can be the best source of advice. There are a lot of people out there who are willing and able to help. Let's suppose you have a problem you require help with. People are more likely to help if you have taken the trouble of providing a very clear picture.

You may find the steps in Fig. 6.1 below worth following.

fig. 6.1 **Eight steps in asking for help from newsgroups**

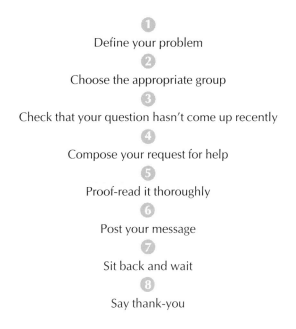

① Define your problem

② Choose the appropriate group

③ Check that your question hasn't come up recently

④ Compose your request for help

⑤ Proof-read it thoroughly

⑥ Post your message

⑦ Sit back and wait

⑧ Say thank-you

Let's take a closer look at the above steps.

① Define your problem

Suppose you have a friend who is in bad shape and needs help. When requesting advice, give as much relevant information as you can. To write to a newsgroup and simply say "My friend is in bad shape and needs help. What can I do?" is hardly going to get you a useful response. However, if you say something like this: "I have a friend who has recently suffered some traumatic life events, and could do with some counselling to help get his life back on track . . . Does anyone know where I can get help?" Defining your problem along that line has more chance of getting a reply. So, before putting together your request, gather as much information as possible about your problem. In the example above the problem is with a friend's health. The kind of information you could gather and add to the problem state are: where does he live; is he able to travel to obtain help; has he got a GP or is there any reason why his GP should not be involved? The definition of the problem should be concise yet clear with all relevant details.

② Choose the appropriate group

It is important that you address your problem to the correct group. In the scenario described previously, any of the following groups may be able to help:

sci.med.nursing
soc.suport.depression.crisis
sci.med.diseases.mental

③ **Check that your question hasn't come up recently**

Look through all available postings from the chosen group and if the group keeps a FAQ, check it to see that your problem isn't in it.

④ **Compose your request for help**

Remember that the people out there are not obliged to help you. A polite request is more likely to produce a positive response.

⑤ **Proof-read it thoroughly**

Check all headers for accuracy, in particular your e-mail address. If it is incorrect, any reply you may get will **bounce**.

⑥ **Post your message**

When you have done all the above, send your e-mail. Make sure you keep a copy for future reference.

⑦ **Sit back and wait**

Once your message is gone, all you can do is to wait. Be patient. Remember that it can take several days before your posting gets round the world.

⑧ **Say thank you**

If you have succeeded in obtaining a helpful reply from anyone, show your gratitude by sending a "thank you" message. It costs nothing and can make people more willing to help you next time.

6.2 getting involved with mailing lists

Mailing lists differ from newsgroups in that a separate copy of the mailing list message is e-mailed to each recipient on the list.

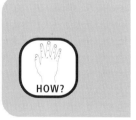

HOW?

A list is set up to discuss a particular topic, and people subscribe to the list. When you send a message to the list, a computer program known as a *list server* (the actual name may be listserv, listproc, majordomo, or one of several other programs) automatically sends it to all the subscribers of the list. Harmon (1996)[14] reports that there are over 6,500 different mailing lists covering a wide range of topics.

6.2.1 mailing addresses

Each mailing list has two addresses. A *List address* and an *Administrative or List Server address*. It is very important that you send your messages to the correct address.

1. **List address** – (Almost) anything sent to the list address is re-mailed to all the people on the list. People on the list respond to messages, creating a running conversation. A reviewer scans some lists and (s)he decides which to send out. Use this address for messages you want distributed to all subscribers on the list.

2. **Administrative address** – Direct your message to this address, if you want it to be read only by the owner of the list. You should always use the administrative address when you are requesting something, such as to:

   ▶ subscribe or unsubscribe from the list;
   ▶ get information about a list;
   ▶ receive a digest version of a list;
   ▶ get a list of request commands;
   ▶ find all the lists on that system.

Some lists are maintained manually and others are maintained automatically by a **list server program**. Here is a list of common list server programs:

   ▶ **LISTSERV** – This is a widely used mail server program. It originated in the USA and is now used at sites throughout the world by people who have set up discussion lists on their local Internet host computer (Tseng, Pulter & Hion, 1996).[15]

   ▶ **Mailbase** – This is popular in the UK and runs many discussion lists from a single site (at the University of Newcastle Upon Tyne).

   ▶ **Majordomo** ⎫
   ▶ **Listproc** ⎬ These are the next three popular mail servers.
   ▶ **Mailserve** ⎭

It is often possible to determine if a list is maintained manually or automatically by examining the message header. The administrative address for a list maintained automatically will contain the name of the list server program and, by way of example, might look like this:

   ▶ LISTSERV@listserv.acsu.buffalo.edu
   ▶ mailbase@mailbase.ac.uk
   ▶ majordomo@interaccess.com
   ▶ Mailserv@ac.dal.ca

Determining an administrative address of a manual list

If you know the *list address* of a list that is maintained manually, then it is relatively easy to figure out the *administrative address*. Just add -request to the list address. For example, if the list address is:

midwife@fensende.com

then the administrative address is almost certainly:

midwife-request@fensende.com

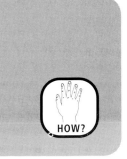

HOW?

6.2.2 finding a mailing list

Almost any list servers will mail you an index of the mailing lists they support. All you need to do is to send them an e-mail message with the word LIST as the body of the message. Here is an example of what e-mail message to send to the server. Fill the **To** field with the list server administrative address then type the following in the **text area**:

LIST GLOBAL / *keyword*

WARNING!

The keyword is the word to look for in list descriptions and names. If you do not add a keyword, you will get a complete list in your e-mail inbox — about 700K of text. Make sure that your service provider can handle that much mail.

You can also visit the five web sites below where you should find excellent indexes and search options to mailing lists:

- http://www.liszt.com
- http:/www.neosoft.com/Internet/pam1/
- http://www.shef.ac.uk/~nhcom
- http://www.tile.net/listserv
- http://www.reference.com/

To get you started, Table 6.4 below offers the administrative addresses of a few mailing lists related to specific topics. For a more comprehensive list, visit any one of the web sites listed above.

table 6.4 **Addresses for mailing lists related to specific topics**

LIST NAME	TO SUBSCRIBE	
and brief description where appropriate	Type this address in the **To** field	Type this message in the **Text area**
ADDICT-L	listserv@kentvm.kent.edu	subscribe addict-l [[YourFirstName] [YourLastName]
AROMA-TRIALS (Related to aromatherapy)	Mailbase@mailbase.ac.uk	subscribe AROMA-TRIALS [YourFirstName] [YourLastName]
CANCER-L	listserv@wvnvm.wvnet.edu	subscribe CANCER-L [YourFirstName] [YourLastName]
CHINs (Community Health Information Networks)	chins-request@chin.net	subscribe chins
CLINICAL FORENSIC NURSING	listserv@ulkyvm.louisville.edu	subscribe ClForNsg [YourFirstName] [YourLastName]

LIST NAME	TO SUBSCRIBE	
CRITCARE	requests@critical-care.co.uk	subscribe critcare
EMERGENCY NURSING	listserv@itssrv1.ucsf.edu	subscribe Em-Nsg-L [YourFirstName] [YourLastName]
HCARENURS (Home Health Nursing Mailing Lists)	majordomo@po.cwru.edu	subscribe HcareNurs [YourE-mailAddress]
HOSPICE	majordomo@po.cwru.edu	subscribe hospice [YourE-mailAddress]
NP-STUDENTS (Nurse Practitioner Listserver)	majordomo@wizards.net	subscribe np-students [YourE-mailAddress]
PNN-L (This is a discussion group for nurse practitioners interested in health promotion, prevention and education)	majordomo@interaccess.com	subscribe PNN-L [YourE-mailAddress]
PSYNURSE	listserv@sjuvm.stjohns.edu	subscribe PSYNURSE [YourFirstName] [YourLastName]
MIDWIFE	midwife-request@fensende.com	Subscribe
AIDS	majordomo@wubios.wustl.edu	Subscribe aids L [YourE-mailAddress]
AUTISM	LISTSERV@utkvm.utk.edu	Subscribe ANI-L [YourFirstName] [YourLastName]
CLICK4HP (Health Promotion)	listserv@yorku.ca	Subscribe click4hp [YourFirstName] [YourLastName]
DEVELOPMENTAL DISABILITIES	LISTSERV@RELAY.ADP.WISC.EDU	Subscribe DDHEALTH
GROUP PSYCHOTHERAPY	listserv@natcom.com	Subscribe Group-Psychotherapy
NURSERES (Nurses Research List)	listserv@listserv.kent.edu	Subscribe NurseRES [YourFirstName] [YourLastName]
NURSE-UK (for nurses interested in UK issues)	majordomo@bham.ac.uk	Subscribe nurse-uk
PEDIATRIC-PAIN	mailserv@ac.dal.ca	Subscribe Pediatric-Pain [YourFirstName] [YourLastName]
DRUGABUS	listserv@umab.umd.edu	sub drugabus [YourFirstName] [YourLastName]
NURSENET (discourse about diverse nursing issues)	listserv@listserv.utoronto.ca	Sub NurseNet [YourFirstName] [YourLastName]
NURSGRAD (This is for the discussion of topics related to graduate nursing education)	listserv@ulkyvm.louisville.edu	Sub NURSGRAD
SNURSE-L (For undergraduate nursing students)	LISTSERV@listserv.acsu.buffalo.edu	Sub Snurse-l [YourFirstName] [YourLastName]
CANCER-NURSING-ALLIANCE	mailbase@Mailbase.ac.uk	join cancer-nursing-alliance [YourFirstName] [YourLastName]
HEALTH-SERVICES-RESEARCH	mailbase@mailbase.ac.uk	join health-services-research [YourFirstName] [YourLastName]
Rogers Theories	mailbase@mailbase.ac.uk	JOIN nurse-rogers [YourFirstName] [YourLastName]
PAEDIATRIC-NURSING-FORUM	mailbase@mailbase.ac.uk	Join paediatric-nursing-forum [YourFirstName] [YourLastName]
PSYCHIATRIC-NURSING (Psychiatric Nursing Discussion Group)	mailbase@mailbase.ac.uk	Join Psychiatric-Nursing [YourFirstName][YourLastName]

Remember that the way you get on or off a mailing list – subscribing or unsubscribing – depends on how the list is maintained ie, whether it is maintained manually or automatically.

For lists that are maintained manually, simply send an e-mail message (like "*please add me to the midwife list*" or "*please remove me from the midwife list*") and send it to the administrative address of that mailing list. The message is read by humans, so no fixed form is required. Do make sure you include your real name.

To subscribe or unsubscribe to a list maintained automatically, you must follow a specific format. Unfortunately, the format that needs to be used to make requests differs slightly from server to server. *Generally* to join a list, you send an e-mail message to its administrative address with nothing written in the *cc, bcc* or *subject fields*, but giving the following basic information in the text area: *List name, your first name, and your last name*. Suppose we wanted to subscribe to 'ADDICT-L', see figure below:

fig. 6.2 **Setting up a subscription to a mailing list**

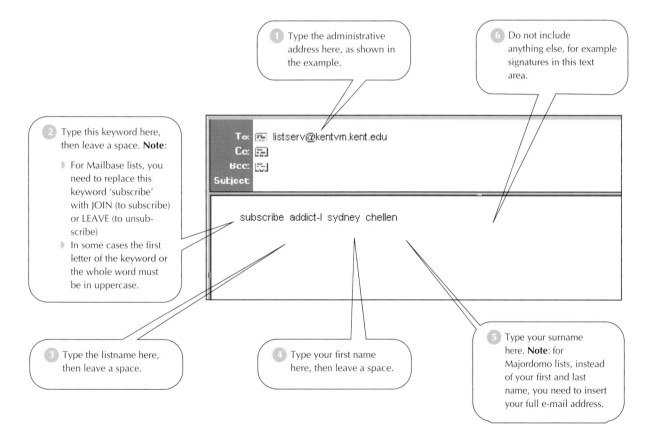

Most, if not all, of the list servers listed in Table 6.4 above will respond to the keyword 'UNSUBscribe' so that you can remove yourself from a list. Send this request to the respective listserver *administrative address*, not the *list address*. For example, for ADDICT-L, address an e-mail to <u>listserv@kentvm.kent.edu</u> and in the text area type: **Unsubscribe addict-l**

When you subscribe to any of the lists mentioned, you will generally be sent a welcome message with instructions for posting to the list, unsubscribing etc – save this message, you will need it later. If you need additional information on how to subscribe to mailing lists you can pay a visit to:

<u>http://www.dundee.ac.uk/~fmsteink/howto.htm</u>

NOTE

Generally you don't need to include your e-mail address because it is automatically included as your message's return address.

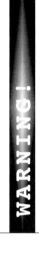

▶ When subscribing to a list, make sure you send your e-mail message from the computer to which you want list messages mailed. This is important, because the administrator of the list uses your message's return address as the address (s)he adds to the mailing list.

▶ Do not subscribe to too many lists at the same time, especially popular lists, as they generate a huge amount of e-mail. You do not want to drown yourself in a deluge of e-mail.

▶ When you know you won't be able to download your e-mail, for example when going on leave, consider unsubscribing from your mailing lists for that period, unless you want to be faced with an overwhelming barrage of e-mail when you log on after your break.

WARNING!

WARNING!

SUBSCRIBING TO A MAILING LIST

activity **6.3**

Using the information given above, select and subscribe to a Mailing list.
If you require additional help please visit this website:
http://www.shef.ac.uk/~nhcon/nulist.htm

When you have completed the activity return to this page and read on

6.2.4 receiving mailing list messages

As soon as you have joined a list, you will automatically receive all messages from the list along with the rest of your e-mail. As some lists are available in *digest* form with all the day's messages combined in a table of contents, you may prefer this digest format. To get the digest form you can send an e-mail message to the list's administrative address with the following lines in the body of the message:

table 6.5 **To receive mailing list messages in digest dormat**

FOR LIST SERVER	TYPE THIS REQUEST IN THE BODY OF YOUR E-MAIL MESSAGE
Listproc	Set <listname> mail digest
LISTSERV	Set <listname> digest
Majordomo	Subscribe <listname> digest, Unsubscribe <listname>
	To undo the digest request
Listproc	Set <listname> mail ack
LISTSERV	Set <listname> mail
Majordomo	Unsubscribe <listname> digest, Subscribe <listname>

6.2.5 sending messages to a mailing list

To send messages to a list that you have subscribed to, you will need to know which computer runs that list (ie, its *list* address – which should be in the details that are returned to you upon subscription). Your message is then automatically distributed to the list's members.

As some lists are screened by a reviewer before being sent off, your message may take a day or two before reaching the members. Good mail servers usually send you copies of your own messages to confirm that they were received. If you have subscribed with Listproc or LISTSERV, you can tell them not to send you copies of your own messages by sending the following message to the administrative address:

table 6.6 **To avoid receiving copies of your own messages**

FOR LIST SERVER	TYPE THIS REQUEST IN THE BODY OF YOUR E-MAIL MESSAGE
Listproc	Set <listname> mail noack
LISTSERV	Set <listname> noack
	To resume receiving copies of your own messages
Listproc	Set <listname> mail ack
LISTSERV	Set<listname> ack

6.2.6 making special requests to mailing lists

After subscribing to a mailing list, there are a few important or desirable requests that you may wish to make. Such as:

- the location of their archive of past messages;
- obtaining a list of all the people who subscribe to the list;
- not wanting your name to be given out to other members.

NOTE

In the <u><listname></u> you need to type the actual name of the list without the smaller (<) or greater (>) signs.

Here is how to do some of them.

To find out where archives of past messages are kept.

Send an e-mail to the administrative address. In the body of the e-mail you should type:

`INDEX <listname>`

> For example, if you subscribe to the Sociology-Midwifery Mailbase List, you can send an e-mail to:
>
> Mailbase@mailbase.ac.uk with the following in the body of the e-mail:
>
> `INDEX sociology-midwifery`

To get a list of all the people who subscribe to a list.

Send an e-mail to the administrative address. In the body of the e-mail you should type the appropriate keyword for that list server:

for list server	type this request in the body of your e-mail message
Listproc	Recipients <listname>
LISTSERV	Review <listname> by name f=mail
Mailbase	Review <listname>
Mailserve	Send <listname>
Majordomo	Who <listname>

To Conceal Your Name

Listproc and LISTSERV won't give your name out by the proceeding process if you send an e-mail to the administrative address.

for list server	type this request in the body of your e-mail message
Listproc	Set <listname> conceal yes
LISTSERV	Set <listname> conceal
To unconceal yourself	
Listproc	Set <listname> conceal no
LISTSERV	Set <listname> noconceal

List servers can do many more tricks. If you want a list of those tricks address an e-mail to <u>LISTSERV@ubvm.cc.buffalo.edu</u> in the body of the e-mail type:

Get mailser cmd nettrain f=mail

6.3 starting an internet relay chat (IRC)

IRC provides real-time conferencing over the Internet. It can be useful for talking to healthcare professionals or students on other continents. However, IRC is not available on all systems, as it tends to use more resources than most system administrators care to devote to it. So, you may find that you cannot use your college network to hold live conversations with others. However, if you have the appropriate system at home you certainly can connect and use this service.

IRC has been described as the CB radio of the Net and it is one of those services that you either love or hate (Hoyler, 1997).[3] You can join one or more "**channels**" (ie, chat rooms) and chat real-time to other healthcare professionals or healthcare students – who can be all over the world. The experience is immediate and can bond you to other people quite quickly.

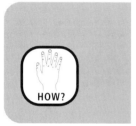

HOW?

With IRC you hold live conversations with others by typing on your keyboard. You type a line or two of text into a small window and press the ENTER key, and the text is almost instantly visible to everyone else taking part. They can respond by typing their own messages, and you'll almost instantly see their responses on your screen. There are now IRC client programs appearing on the market, which allow a bit more of point-and-click approach.

NOTE

In the Internet world, <u>Chatting</u> and <u>Talking</u> are not the same things. But one thing they have in common is their immediacy.

'Chatting' usually takes place in a chat room, which may contain just two or three people, or as many as fifty. Sometimes, no one seems to talk at all. Sometimes two or three conversations are going on between little groups of people, with all messages appearing in the same window, and things can get a bit confusing. Although there may be several people in the room, many are just 'listening' rather than joining in.

'Talking' is a little different. Although the method of sending messages to and fro is the same, 'talk' usually takes place between just two people, and in a more structured way.

HOW?

Using a *talk program*, you'd usually enter the e-mail address of the person you want to talk to, and if that person is online, the conversation begins.

To cloud the issue a bit, *chat programs* also allow two people to enter a private room and 'talk', and many talk programs will allow more people to join in with your conversation if you allow them to enter. This has somewhat smeared the boundary between chat and talk. To complicate things even more, with the recent arrival of

Voice on the Net (VON), you can talk to others using microphones (see section 6.4).

6.3.1 connecting to IRC

The Internet Relay Chat, is the Internet's own chat system. You can connect to it using *Telnet* (for more information see Unit 7, Section 7.4). If you are a beginner you may find that a better approach is to use a piece of software called mIRC. You can download a copy of this program from http://www.mirc.co.uk

To use IRC you first have to connect to your nearest IRC server. There are IRC servers all over the Internet and you can connect to whichever IRC server you want, but you'll get better performance if you choose one close to you. In the UK, the best one to use is **irc.demon.co.uk** run by Demon Internet. If you have a computer system at home with the Internet facility, then do the activity below – it will help you get started.

USING MIRC TO CHAT AND TALK   activity **6.4**

Unless you've already got mIRC installed on your machine, before doing this activity you must first get on the Net, download and install mIRC on your computer. Then, use the program to get connected to an IRC server so that you can start a live conversation.

When you have completed the activity return to this page and read on
If you don't want to or can't do this *activity, read on*

6.3.2 some IRC commands

There are a huge number of commands that you can master and put to use. The mIRC program even includes a general IRC help-file, which explains how they work. A selected few are listed in Table 6.7 to get you started.

It is very easy to use the commands listed previously. Here is a quick example. Suppose you have been holding a chat. You have decided to stop and feel the need to explain why. You can enter this command **/quit Got a lecture to attend. See you tomorrow.**

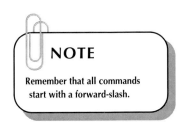

NOTE

Remember that all commands start with a forward-slash.

table 6.7 **A selection of useful IRC commands**

TYPE THIS	TO DO THIS
/help	Get general help on IRC
/list	List all the channels available on the server you are connected to
/list -min n	List all the channels with at least n people in them (replace n with a figure)
/join #channel	Enter a channel. Replace channel with the name of your chosen channel
/leave #channel	Leave the specified channel (or the channel in the current window if no channel is specified)
/quit message	Finish your IRC session and display a message to the channel if you enter one (see below)
/away message	Tell other occupants you're temporarily away from your computer, giving a message
/away	With no message, means that you're no longer away
/whois nickname	Get information about the specified nickname in the main window

6.4 hearing your voice on the net

Voice on the Net (VON) is the latest addition to the Net. It is the Internet equivalent to the telephone. You can hold live conversations with anyone in the world, provided the person is online and has their VON software running.

HOW?

You start the VON program, choose the e-mail address of the person you want to converse with, as soon as the link is established you can start speaking into a microphone. You will hear their responses through your speakers or a headset.

This is a very cost-effective way of holding a conversation with someone far away. Suppose you are in the UK and want to converse with someone in New Zealand, you simply dial into your local access provider, paying only a local telephone call, even though you are speaking to someone abroad. Apart from this, you can send computer files back and forth, hold conferences, or even use a whiteboard to draw sketches and diagrams. However, as both you and the person you are calling must be online, both of you will pay telephone charges. Despite this downside, the combined cost could still amount to less than 10% of a conventional international call charge. Some recent systems allow you to dial someone's telephone number rather than e-mail address, making it possible to make these cheap international calls to someone who doesn't even have their own Internet account.

Currently, you must be using the same VON program as the other person you want to converse with. If you have several people you want to talk to, you may need to have several different VON programs installed on your computer. Fortunately, some VON programs are free. The situation is bound to change.

CHECKLIST OF HARDWARD SPECIFICATIONS

activity **6.5**

VON programs have some definite hardware specifications. Use this check-list to tick (✓) your requirements.

○ A sound card (preferably **full-duplex** card),
○ A fairly fast computer eg, a Pentium
○ 8Mb RAM or more,
○ A microphone and speakers plugged into your sound card,
○ A modem: 28.8Kbps or higher connected to a phone line,
○ VON software

> **TECHNO TALK**
> A full-duplex card can record your voice while playing the incoming voice. This enables both of you to talk at the same time (ideal for discussions). With half-duplex you can either talk or listen, but not both.

6.4.1 a selection of VON programs

There is a wide selection of VON programs to choose from. Here is a short list:

1. **Internet Phone** A VON program that you will need to pay for, otherwise your talk time will be limited. You can obtain and register an evaluation copy at http://www.vocaltec.com

2. **NetMeeting** A Microsoft VON program. You can download a free copy from http://www.microsoft.com/netmeeting

3. **PowWow** A very user-friendly program and it is free. You can download it from http://www.tribal.com

4. **Web Phone** A very stylish VON program. For an evaluation copy visit http://www.itelco.com

summary and conclusion

Newsgroups form an important part of the Internet. Getting involved in these can be an interesting and informative way of trading information. A more personal manner of communicating is with mailing lists. Both of those methods can prove to be useful sources of information and the people involved in the newsgroups may be able to solve your problems. If you want a faster medium then try IRCs. These can also prove useful but also quite expensive if done from a home PC.

the gateway to free health and medical resources

> "I used to have to drive 30 miles to get to my college library, only to discover that the books I need are out or unavailable. Now, from the comfort of my own home I can telnet into my library computer, browse through their catalogues and order the books I want. All with a few clicks of my mouse."
>
> *A part-time BSc student*

Although e-mail and the web will probably meet most of your needs, there are additional tools that you will hear mentioned which can help you use your browser more effectively. They were around long before the World Wide Web started dominating the Internet.

Four of these are **FTP**, **Archie**, **Gopher** and **Telnet**. The functions of many of these tools are now performed by web browsers like NetScape Navigator or Microsoft Internet Explorer. However, there may be occasions when it is necessary for you to use these tools directly to gain access to all those millions of computers around the world. For example, you may become aware of statistics that support a project you are completing, a computer program that can help you perform your health data analysis, or documents that offer a bibliography for a course assignment. With the right privilege you can grab these files and transfer them to your computer free of charge. Or you may need to quickly search a computerised library catalogue to find available material to complete a project, but do not wish to trot from library to library. In this unit, the four tools mentioned above will be discussed. It includes explanation on how to use them to find what you want, and where appropriate how to download your find to your hard disk.

TECHNOTALK

FTP stands for File Transfer Protocol. It is a method of transferring files from one computer to another over the Net.

Archie is an older system that was and can still be used to find files that are located on the FTP sites.

Gopher is an older system that lets you find text information by using menus.

Telnet is a system that lets you connect from your computer to another across the Internet and use it as if you were directly connected to that computer. A slightly different version of telnet, developed by *IBM*, is known as tn3270.

checklist

Below is a checklist of what you can expect to find out in this Unit. Read through the statements then tick (✓) the items about which you would like to know more.

I would like to find out more about:

Please turn over the page and read through the topics you have ticked

FTP stands for File Transfer Protocol. It is a method of transferring files from one computer to another over the Net. It works in a similar way to *File Manager* (on Windows 3.1 and NT) and *Windows Explorer* on Windows 95/98. While with File Manager or Windows Explorer you can open directories, browse around and copy any file to another directory on your hard disk or floppy disk, with FTP you can copy files from another computer to your own or vice versa.

While completing Units 2, 3 and 4 you have already made some use of FTP without perhaps realising it. You may recall while surveying web pages you have been clicking on **links**. These links were letting you download files. Some of these files were stored on web servers and others on FTP servers. Next time you surf the Net, and you come to a link, simply rest your mouse-pointer on the link and look at your browser's status-bar. If the link is pointing to an FTP site, you will see the address starts with **ftp://**

The addresses (URLs) of FTP sites look almost like web addresses – they begin with the type of server (computer) and continue with the directory path to the specific file. Here is a quick comparison of the two URLs. Notice that one starts with *http://* and the other starts with *ftp://*

A web URL: http://www.diabetic.org.uk/index.htm

An ftp URL: ftp://ftp.liv.ac.uk/pub/epidemic/

Before exploring how to get into FTP sites, let's first clarify the difference between private and anonymous sites.

7.1.1 private vs anonymous sites

Some FTP sites hold confidential files and, therefore, only those with special privileges can access them. They are known as private FTP sites. Many other sites, known as **anonymous** FTP sites, give free access to all their files. However, some of these anonymous sites may only have their top-level directory called pub or public which contain non-confidential files. In which case, only the public can access these non-confidential files.

Whether you are trying to access a private or anonymous site you will need a *username* and a *password* to log in, just as you do when you connect to your service provider's system.

If you had a special account with privileges to access confidential files on a private or anonymous site, when you log in the computer will recognise who you are by your username and password. In this Unit we are going to concern ourselves with access to anonymous sites that are open to the public.

How to get access to FTP sites

To get access to FTP sites you simply connect your computer to an FTP server — an Internet host computer that stores files for transfer. To make this connection you can use one of the following:

▸ your browser,
▸ a real FTP program, or
▸ your e-mail program.

In the next three sections, all the above will be discussed.

HOW?

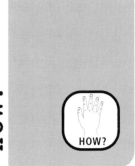

7.1.2 using your browser to access ftp sites

You can use Microsoft Internet Explorer, NetScape Navigator (or any other browsers) to access non-confidential files at any anonymous FTP sites. As the two browsers mentioned above are so sophisticated, you won't be prompted to enter anything. The browser will handle everything automatically for you. The activity below will show you how easy it is to use Internet Explorer (or NetScape Navigator) to access a file on an FTP site.

USING YOUR BROWSER TO ACCESS FTP SITES   activity **7.1**

Let's suppose you're looking for the *Liverpool School of Tropical Medicine Meningitis Epidemic Case Study*. You have been told that the file is called **epidemic** and it is located at this URL: ftp://ftp.liv.ac.uk/pub/epidemic/

Using the knowledge and skills you have or have acquired from previous units in this book, go and get this file. (*Clue*: log on to Windows and start your browser. Type the URL in the **Location/Address** box, then press the RETURN key. Provided there is no problem, the requested page should appear on your screen.

When you have completed the activity return to this page and read on

The above activity was not too difficult I hope. You may have noticed that it was no different to searching for a known file on the web, except that you had to go to an FTP site to locate it. The next section will discuss the second method of obtaining files from FTP sites.

7.1.3 using a dedicated ftp program

As you begin to get more acquainted with the Internet, you may want more control over the file transfer process – especially, when later on you create your own web site and you want to copy files to your access provider's web server. In this case, you would find a 'real' FTP program more user-friendly, and sometimes it will connect to an FTP site faster than a browser can. A dedicated FTP program also gives you more information about the progress of downloads from FTP sites than a browser does. There are several FTP programs that you can use. Here are two of the best FTP programs around currently:

▶ **WS_FTP LE for Windows** A very popular program. You can find the fully-fledged WS_FTP Professional including updates at this web site: http://www.ipswitch.com

▶ **FTP Explorer** A nice little program designed for Windows95 and later. For a version of it look at http://www.ftpx.com

When you use FTP programs like those described above, you simply click on the label **Anonymous** and all necessary details will be entered for you. You may find that your college/university has one of these FTP programs – or a similar one – already installed on the network.

If you have Internet access at home, you may wish to install it on your system. To do this, pay a visit to the web sites given above and grab a copy of WS_FTP or FTP Explorer. You should find on-screen instruction on how to download the program. Installing WS_FTP is simplicity itself. Activity 7.2 offers some assistance.

activity 7.2   USING A DEDICATED FTP PROGRAM TO ACCESS FTP SITES

You only need to carry out this activity if you would like to use one of the two FTP programs mentioned previously, on your home system, with a view to surfing FTP sites.

▶ Log on to the Internet (using your home or college system) and enter the URL http://www.ipswich.com in the **Address/Location** box of your browser. Once you are at the web site containing the WS_FTP program, follow the on-screen instructions and download it to a floppy disk.

▶ Following the instructions in **Worksheet 11**, create a 'Session Profile' that will connect you to an FTP site in WS_FTP.

▶ Now, using the WS_FTP program, see if you can replicate the activity in 7.1.

When you have completed the activity return to p. 149 and read on

worksheet **11**

SETTING UP WS_FTP

① Start WS_FTP. *As this is your first session, you will be asked to enter your e-mail address. Once you have done so, the Session Properties dialogue box (shown below) should appear.*

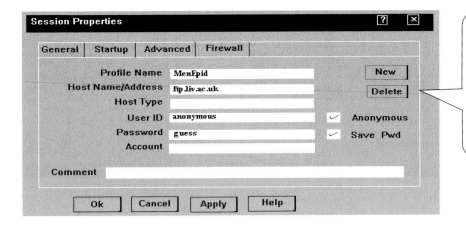

② Point and click on the button labelled New.

③ In the **Profile Name** box, you can type any name to help you identify a site in the future. For our purpose type **MenEpid**

④ In the **Host Name/Address** box, type the name of the computer you want to connect to. For our purpose type **ftp.liv.ac.uk**

⑤ You can ignore the Host type box. WS_FTP will work it out for you.

⑥ As we are connecting to an anonymous FTP site, point and click the **Anonymous** box. *This will place a checkmark in it.* (If you were going to a private site, you would have needed to type your username in the **User ID** box.)

⑦ As we are entering an anonymous site, type **guess** in the **Password** box. (If you're visiting a private site, you will have typed your password. Also, if you don't want to enter your password each time you visit this site, you point and click on the Save Pwd to place a checkmark in it.)

⑧ Point and click the **Startup** tab. In the box labelled **Initial Remote Host Directory**, type the path to the directory you want to start in when connected. For our purpose type **/pub/epidemic/** (don't forget that very first forward slash).

⑨ In the box marked **Initial Local Directory**, you can type the path to a directory on your own computer that you want any files to be downloaded. For our purpose type **a:**
   Note: Every time you connect to this site drive a: will be selected.

10 Point and click on the **OK** button. *WS_FTP will save these settings for future use and try to connect to the site when requested.*

If you have completed the activity above, did you find any difference between the two methods of searching for a file on FTP sites?

The third method of reaching FTP sites is by using e-mail program. This is equally simple. All you need is to have a facility to send and receive e-mail.

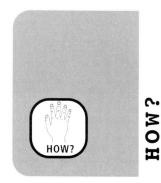

Using an e-mail program to get to FTP sites

If you have only e-mail access to the Internet you need not worry as you can still obtain the benefits of FTP. To access anonymous sites using your e-mail program, you simply log in with the username <u>anonymous</u> and give your e-mail address, or the word <u>guess</u>, as your password. Unfortunately, this versatility comes at a cost, can be tricky to manage, and first-time success is the exception rather than the rule (McKenzie, 1995).[16] For further information on transferring files using e-mail read McKenzie's book, Unit 19, pp 143–7.

7.2 using archie to find the health material you want

NOTE

'Archie' happens to be a famous cartoon character. The names of two other characters – 'Veronica' and 'Jughead' – from the same cartoon have been used to label two other search systems.

Archie servers are located around the Internet. They can help you find the exact location of the files you are looking for literally in seconds. These servers keep track of all the anonymous FTP public files on the Internet by searching the public directories of the FTP hosts on a regular basis and maintaining a list of all files.

If you know what file you want and where to get it, then there is usually no big problem, as you would have already found out when you carried out Activities 7.1 and 7.2. However, the difficulty comes when you only have part of the information needed, then obtaining what you want may not be that easy at first. Take this scenario:

Suppose you have heard of a file or program that may help you with a particular health assignment you are researching, and luckily enough someone has told you the name and location of that file/program.

In the scenario above there is no problem: you simply type the URL into your browser's location box (like you did in activities 7.1 and 7.2) and look for the file when the directory's contents are shown. But what if you only knew the location and not the name of the file? Then it is a bit like searching for a needle in a haystack. You could go to that location, enter the directory and view or download one of the Index files. This usually gives a short description of each file in that directory. With a bit of luck you might find the file you want.

However, if you knew the name of the file, and didn't know its location, the situation is much more promising but you may not necessarily want to spend hours searching computers. This is when you will appreciate what *Archie* can do for you. You can either use Archie on the web or a dedicated Archie program to connect to one of the **Archie servers**. Here are two of the best dedicated Archie programs:

▶ **wsArchie** This program is the other half of the WS_FTP program mentioned earlier. For a free copy, visit this web site:
http://dspace.dial.pipex.com/town/square/cc83

▶ **fpArchie** This program is even better because it does not need a separate FTP program. When it locates the file, it will download it for you. For a free copy of this program, visit this web site:
http://www.euronet.nl/~petert/fpware

Now try the activity below. It is designed to help you experience using Archie.

USING ARCHIE TO FIND A FILE   activity **7.3**

In Activity 7.1 you had all the essential information you needed, therefore you were able to locate the file: *'meningitis epidemic case study'*.

This time let's pretend that you only know the name of the file and nothing else. See if you can use *Archie on the web* or a *dedicated Archie program* to find it.

Do enlist someone on the Helpdesk to help you identify the *Archie program icon* on your college system. Activate it, then try to find the file mentioned above.
or

If you are connect to the Internet at home, visit one of the websites mentioned above and download *wsArchie* or *fpArchie*. Install the program on your computer system. Then try using it to find the file.

When you have completed the activity return to this page and read on

How did you get on using Archie?

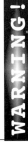

```
Although all Archie servers do much the same job, some find files that others
don't. If a search ends in no results, choose a different server from the
picklist of wsArchie's or fpArchie's drop-down menu. If you are unable to get
to a particular Archie server because it is too busy, try again later.
```

WARNING!

7.3 'gopherspace'

Prior to the World Wide Web, the Gopher system was the friendly face of the Internet. It is an older Internet filing system that presents information as a series of menus. It consists of a number of computers around the world acting as Gopher servers (just as there are web servers, news servers, FTP servers and so on).

In Units 2&3, you were encouraged to explore the World Wide Web, and look at documents stored on web servers. In this section, you will be offered some information on connecting to Gopher servers and getting into 'Gopherspace' to search for documents.

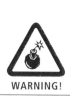

NOTE

Before attempting to access gopher sites on your college system, you should check with the Computing department whether it has a gopher client installed on the system.

For any Gopher sites that you come across, you should find that your web browser should enable you to access them. Recognising Gopher sites is easy, as they have URLs that start with **gopher://**, for example: Gopher://gopher.tc.umn.edu, which is the gopher of the University of Minnesota. Simply type the gopher URL in your browser's location box and provided it is properly configured you should be transported to your chosen site.

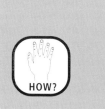

HOW?

HOW?

How does a Gopher work?

The Gopher server can be anywhere on the Internet. When you select an item on a menu, your service provider's computer sends a message to the remote gopher telling it to send you that item. The process is similar to you requesting a catalogue from a company; you select an item from the catalogue, and then the company posts the chosen item to you. The difference is that with gopher you do not get a bill at the end of the month.

If you are unable to access Gopher sites on your college system, and you are desperate to do so, you can always install a dedicated Gopher program like *wsGopher* on your home system. For more information, pay a visit to:

http://www.mstc.com

Connections between gophers are seamless, so you can move from one gopher to another without realising it. You can retrieve text information from different parts of the world with equal ease.

Before we had Windows and mice, to use a computer you had to type commands from the keyboard. When the Internet became available for general use, people wanted to operate a computer at a distance; this gave birth to a service called Telnet. Although the Telnet service has been eclipsed by the flexibility of the World Wide Web, there are places you can only get to via Telnet. For example, if you want to log in and access your college/university computerised library catalogue from home, you will need Telnet to open a command line connection to their library computer.

The simplicity of Telnet makes it look boring. You get a command line, no graphics, and no sound (except for the occasional beep). However, the benefits are that it is simple to use and from the comfort of your home you can connect to your college library catalogue to:

- Search the library catalogue;

- Reserve any items out on loan;

- Check your own borrower record and renew items;

- Place inter-library loans.

This saves you the hassle of paying a bus fare or driving to your institution to find out if it has the books you want for your assignments. However, don't expect to be able to actually read the books online – maybe one day!

To use Telnet, you need a Telnet software installed on your PC, or your web browser set up to handle Telnet calls. As Telnet is not a growing service, there are a limited number of Telnet programs around. Ewan is by far the best Telnet program. However, if you are using Windows 95 or 98, then you already have a good Telnet program incorporated and ready for use. To learn how to use it try Activity 7.4.

SEARCHING LIBRARY CATALOGUES FROM HOME   **activity 7.4**

This activity will take you through the process of using your Windows 95 or 98 program to connect to the online library catalogue of: *Canterbury Christ Church University College*. Follow the step-by-step instructions listed in **Worksheet 12**.

Carry out a search. Use the steps in **Worksheet 13** to printout your search results.

When you have completed the activity return to p. 154 and read on

To connect to your library computer system you can use a dedicated Telnet program like *Ewan* or if you have Windows95 or 98 installed on your home system, you can use the built in Telnet program.

CONNECTING TO A COMPUTERISED LIBRARY SYSTEM

1. Start **Windows95** or **98**

2. Click on **Start** button. *A menu should pop-up.*

3. Click on the command **Run**. *A run dialogue box should appear.*

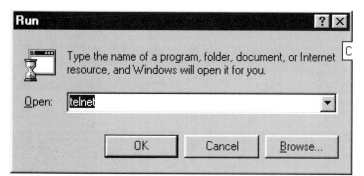

4. Type **Telnet** and then press the **ENTER** key. *A Telnet window should appear.*

5. Click on the command **Connect**. *A sub-menu should drop-down.*

6. Click on the command **Remote System**. *A Connect dialogue box should appear.*

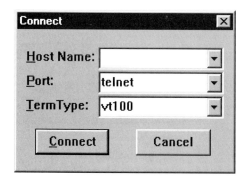

7. Type the site's address in the **Host Name** box

To connect to
Canterbury Christ Church University College
you should type:
Gateway.cant.ac.uk.

And click on the **Connect** button

8. Now dial your Service Provider, entering the appropriate information required. *After a moment you should be connected to the library. When the library window appears, wait until you see a 'Telnet gateway' prompt. (Warning: This may take a while.)*

9. At the "Telnet gateway" prompt, type **connect library** then press the ENTER key.

10. To log in, type the username which is **library** then press the ENTER key. *You should now be in. When you want to leave the library catalogue, type **Exit** and press the **ENTER** key.*

Note: If you experience any problems, please contact your Internet Service Provider for Help and advice on your computer set-up.

PRINTING YOUR SEARCH RESULTS

To print, you will need to copy and paste your results into a word-processing package, by following the instructions below:

1. From **Edit** menu, choose **Select All** to copy the whole screen or drag and highlight selected areas.

2. From the **Edit** menu, choose **Copy**.

3. Open word-processing package, eg, word.

4. From the **Edit** menu, choose **Paste**.

5. For a print out, click on the print icon located on the toolbar of your wordprocessor.

Virtually all university libraries in the UK have a computerised catalogue, and the vast majority of these are accessible via the Internet. The same is also true for foreign universities. You can find a listing of UK and US libraries at:

http://www.cam.ac.uk/Hytelnet/uk0/uk000.html
http://library.usask.ca/hytelnet/

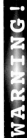

Public libraries are slower in connecting to the Internet. The British Library has its own online service, but in order to use the catalogue you will need to register. This will cost you a yearly fee. For more details go to the following website:

http://portico.bl.uk/

WARNING!

summary and conclusion

Besides e-mail and WWW, there are additional tools such as FTP, Archie, Gopher and Telnet to help you get the best out of the Internet. For example, FTPs can be immensely helpful with your research project. You will also find that when you are in need of help finding the location of some pieces of information, Archie can do wonders for you. Finally with the right hardware and software at home you can telnet your way into your institute's library in the comfort of your home.

publishing on the world wide web

"I found it personally rewarding to design my first homepage, and then to upload it successfully to my Internet Service Provider. But the real satisfaction came when I was able to visit the site and view my efforts." Newall (1999)[17]

Senior Lecturer Nursing Studies
Canterbury Christ Church University College, Canterbury.
Faculty of Nursing and Social Work.
http://www.enewall.free-online.co.uk

Now that you have learnt about the most essential services on the Net and how to use them, they remain the creation of others. Having your own homepage is one of the best ways of publishing your ideas and creations to the world. You will find many service providers are keen and ready to enable you to create and maintain a homepage as part of your basic account. The mechanics of creating a web page are amazingly simple. In this unit, following an explanation of the most important component parts of a webpage, you should be able to create a simple web page of your own.

checklist

Below is a checklist of what you can expect to find out in this Unit. Read through the statements then tick (✓) the items about which you would like to know more.

I would like to find out more about:

Please turn over the page and read through the topics you have ticked

HTML (HyperText Markup Language) is the language used to create web pages. The markup language is a set of codes or signs added to plain text to indicate how it should be presented to the reader, taking into consideration bold, italic or underlined text, typefaces to be used, beginning and ending of paragraphs, etcetera, etcetera, etcetera.

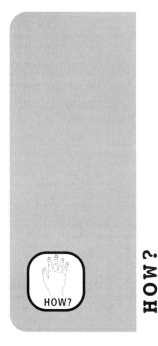

How does HTML work?

Suppose you were using a word processor — like Word for Windows — to type a document, and you wanted a particular text in a sentence to appear in bold. To get the bold effect you simply highlight the desired text and click on the bold icon. You do not have to worry about the codes that make the word appear in bold. The word processor takes care of this for you and hides them from your view.

However, when you prepare a document to be displayed as a webpage, and you wanted a particular text to appear in bold, you will need to type the appropriate code along with the text like this:

<B>This is bold</B> and this is plain

When the browser displays the webpage containing that text, it uses the codes to show the bold feature like this:

This is bold and this is plain

Likewise, it uses other codes that you insert to show other features.

Tags are the *HTML* codes added to plain text in a document. This transforms it into a web page with full formatting and links to other files and pages.

These codes are known as **tags** and they consist of ordinary text placed between the less-than and greater-than signs. In the example above, the first tag, <B>, means 'turn on bold type'. Halfway through the sentence a second tag, </B>, is used meaning 'turn off bold type'. Notice that to turn off bold, the same tag is used again, but with a forward-slash inserted immediately after the less-than sign. There are several other codes, a few of which you need to be familiar with. Those codes are so logical that you should have no trouble remembering them. See Table 8.1 for a selected list.

To create a web page you need two of the following tools:

- a homepage wizard, or
- a web page editor like Internet Assistant for Word for Windows, or
- a text editor like Windows NotePad, or
- any word processor which can store text in ascii format,
- **plus** a web browser to test out your pages and to get you on to the Internet.

table 8.1 **Formatting tags and their functions. A tag is distinguished from the rest of the text by being surrounded by < >.**

<HTML>	Use the tag on the left to indicate the beginning of a file, and use the one on the right to indicate the end of the file.	</HTML>
<HEAD>	Use the left and right tags to indicate the beginning and ending of a heading section.	</HEAD>
<TITLE>	Use the left and right tags to surround the title of the page.	</TITLE>
<BODY>	Use the left tag at the start of your content of the page and use the right tag to indicate the end of the content.	</BODY>
<B>	Use the left and right tags to turn on and off bold.	</B>
<I>	Use the left and right tags to turn on and off italic.	</I>
<U>	Use the left and right tags to turn on and off underlining.	</U>
<Hn>	There are six heading tags <H1> </H1> to <H6> </H6>. The text enclosed between the heading tags appears in that style. <H1> is the most prominent heading style. Use the left and right tags to surround a level n heading, where 'n' stands for a number.	</Hn>
<FONT size=number>	Use this tag to state the size of the font. Number=1–7.	</font>
 	Use the tag on the left to indicate a line break. It does not need a closing tag.	
<P>	Use the left and right tags to split text into paragraphs.	</P>
<HR>	Use the tag on the left to draw a horizontal line across the page. This tag also causes a line break.	
<A HREF="*linkname*"> *texttolink*	Use the left tag to link your page to another web site. Replace the *linkname* by the URL of the web site you want to link to and replace the *texttolink* by a keyword or keyphrase.	</A>
<img src="URL">	Use this tag to display an image.	
<Centre>	Use the left and right to put text in the centre of a line.	</centre>

STEPS FOR CREATING A SIMPLE WEB PAGE — activity 8.1

▶ Using Windows Notepad create a template and then use it to create a web page. For help on doing this, please follow the instructions in **Worksheet 14**.

▶ Now view your creation using your Browser. For help on how to do this, follow the instructions listed in **Worksheet 15**.

When you have completed the activity return to p. 160 and read on

NOTE

There are certain basic *tags* that will appear in almost every *HTML* document. We can start by making a 'template file' that we can use every time we want to create a new page. I will assume that you are using the Notepad program available in Windows.

Comment

None of these tags do anything exciting by themselves but are very important in the construction of the web page. Your document has to be placed between the <HTML> and the </HTML> tags.
There are two chunks: the **head** (the section between <HEAD> and </HEAD>) and the **body** (between <BODY> and </BODY>).

The head will contain the title inserted between the <TITLE> and </TITLE> tags and the body will contain the text you want to appear on your webpage, and this will be typed between the <BODY> and </BODY> tags.

The body will also contain tags you need to display images, set colours, hyperlinks to other pages and sites and other things you want on your page.

CREATING A TEMPLATE

1. Start Notepad

2. Now, type the text below:

```
<HTML>
<HEAD>
<TITLE>Untitled</TITLE>
</HEAD>

<BODY>

</BODY>
</HTML>
```

3. (For the purpose of this exercise) save this file to a **floppy disk** as **myweb1.htm**

USING THE TEMPLATE TO CREATE A WEB PAGE

1. Replace the word **Untitled** with a suitable title for the document, for example **My homepage**.

2. Now add some text to the page. You can copy what I have done below or replace it with your own entries.

3. When you've completed that, insert a formatted floppy disk in drive A.

4. Save the file to the **floppy disk** as **myweb2.htm**.

```
<HTML>
<HEAD>
<TITLE>My homepage</TITLE>
</HEAD>

<BODY>
<H1>Welcome! </H1>
This is my first attempt at creating a webpage.
<P> I hope you like it. </P>
</BODY>
</HTML>
```

DISPLAYING YOUR CREATION

1 Ensure the floppy disk on which you saved the file **myweb2.htm** is in drive A.

2 Open your Browser (You do not need to be *online*).

3 Choose the command **File** on the menubar. *A submenu should drop-down.*

4 Choose the command **Open**. *An Open dialog box should appear, and the cursor should be flashing in a white rectangular box.*

5 Type **a:\myweb2.htm** then click the **OK** button. *Your Browser should display your creation, which should look like the screenshot below.*

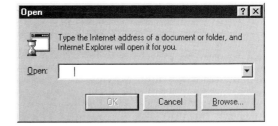

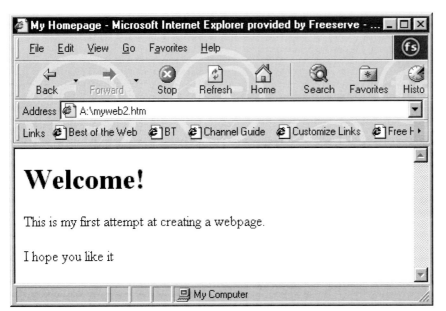

8.2.1 maximising html

Although the web page you have created in the activity above is a simple one, it is just as easy to spice up that page by changing text size and font, adding links to other web pages, adding colour and background, and even pictures.

For example, if you want to make your text **Bold**, *Italic* or <u>Underlined</u>, or all three, you simply surround the text with the appropriate tags like this:

I want to be <B>bold</B>. No, I prefer to be in <I>italic</I>. No, I want to be <U>underlined</U>. I really want to be <B><I><U>bold, italic and underlined</B></I></U>.

This is how your browser will display the above:

I want to be **bold**. No I prefer to be in *italic*. No I want to be <u>underlined</u>. I really want to be ***<u>bold, italic and underlined</u>***.

Since the tags <B> for bold, <I> for italic and <U> for underline have ongoing effects, you need to enter the closing tags </B>, </I>, and </U> to stop the effects.

There are six heading tags that change the size of the text. <H1> is the most prominent heading style and <H6> is the least prominent.

For example:
<H1> Welcome! </H1>

Welcome!

<H6> Welcome! </H6>
Welcome!

You can also use the *font tag* to change the font size. Sizes range from 1 to 7, with 1 being the smallest and 7 being the largest.

For example:
<FONT SIZE=3> My homepage </FONT>

My homepage

The <BR> tag provides a line break without adding a line space.

For example:

Welcome to . . .
 My homepage!

Welcome to . . .
My homepage!

The <P> tag also ends a line, but adds a line space. You should use this to split text into paragraphs.

For example:

Welcome to . . . <P> My homepage!

Welcome to . . .

My homepage!

The <HR> tag divides the page into sections by drawing a horizontal line across the page. It also causes a line break.

For example:

Mental Health Act:

<HR>

Section 2 – Admission for assessment

<HR>

Section 3 – Admission for treatment

<HR>

Section 4 – Emergency admission for assessment

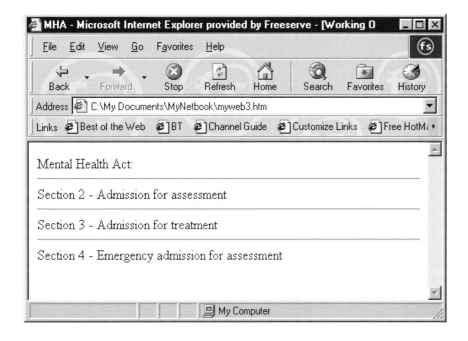

The hallmark of a web site is that it should contain links to other web sites. You can use link tags to add a *hyperlink* to other web pages. The tag is:

<A HREF= "*link name*"> *texttolink* </A>

For example:

Suppose you want to create a link from your webpage (ie, the one you created while doing Activity 8.1) to, say, the UK Department of Health webpage. You can start a new paragraph and add the following:

<P> For more information visit the <A HREF= "
http://www.open.gov.uk/doh/dhhome.htm"> *Dept. of Health* </A> *site.*

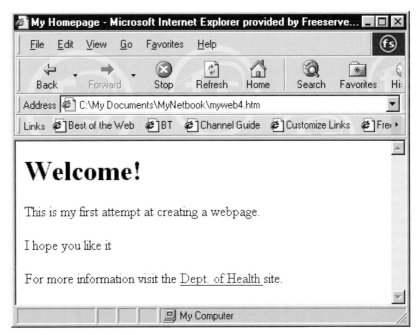

The screenshot above shows the result. The next activity will help you add this link to your page. First, here is additional explanation about the link tag.

In HTML the link tags are referred to as 'anchors'. That's what the A after the first < sign means. An opening anchor usually begins with this tag: <A HREF= "*link name*">.

Instead of the *link name* you type the URL of the page you want to link to, in between the quotation marks.

Immediately after the > sign, where it says *texttolink*, you type in a keyword or keyphrase that you want visitors to your page to click on. Finally, type in the closing anchor tag, </A>.

It is assumed that you have completed Activity 8.1 and you saved your work using the filenames instructed.

Follow the instructions in **Worksheets 16 and 17**. You will be shown how to use the 'Link tag' to link your web page to another web site.

When you have completed the activity return to p. 166 and read on

CREATING A LINK TO ANOTHER WEB SITE (1)   **worksheet 16**

ADDING A LINK ON YOUR WEB PAGE

1. Start Notepad.

2. Insert in **Drive A** the floppy disk containing the file **myweb2.htm**

3. Click the command **File** on the menubar. *A submenu should appear.*

4. Click on the command **Open**. *An Open dialog box should appear.*

5. In the Filename box type: **A:\myweb2.htm** then press **ENTER**. *The document you prepared earlier should now be loaded into Notepad.*

6. Now, modify the document so that it contains all the lines as shown below:

```
<HTML>
<HEAD>
<TITLE>My homepage </TITLE>
</HEAD>
<BODY>
<H1> Welcome! </H1>
This is my first attempt at creating a webpage.
<P> I hope you like it </P>
<P> For more information visit the
<A HREF="http://www.open.gov.uk/doh/dhhome.htm">
Dept. of Health </A> site.
</BODY>
</HTML>
```

7. For the purpose of this exercise save this file back to your **floppy disk** as **myweb3.htm**

DISPLAYING YOUR NEW WEBPAGE

1. Ensure the floppy disk on which you saved the file **myweb3.htm** is in drive A.

2. Open your Browser (You do not need to be *online*).

3. Choose the command **File** on the menubar. *A submenu should drop-down.*

4. Choose the command **Open**. *An Open dialog box should appear, and the cursor should be flashing in a white rectangular box.*

5. Type **a:\myweb3.htm** then press ENTER. *Your Browser should display your new webpage containing the link to the Department of Health, as shown in the screenshot below.*

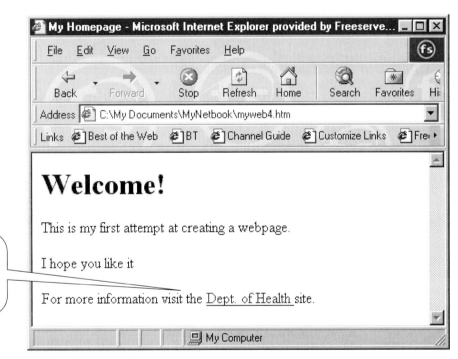

Comment

If you point and click on the Keyphrase: *Dept. of Health*, your browser should take you that site.

Another type of anchor allows a visitor to your page to e-mail you from their web browsers. As the person clicks the link, it opens their e-mail message window, with your e-mail address already inserted, ready for them to send you a message. Suppose I wanted to create a link on my web page so that visitors can e-mail me, here is how I will do it:

<A HREF="mailto:s.s.chellen@cant.ac.uk">Click here to send me an e-mail </A>

As you can see I have replaced the URL with my e-mail address and I have also inserted the word **mailto:** immediately after that first quote sign. To do the same to your web page, simply replace my e-mail address with yours.

Another good way to spice up your web page is to add images. You will find lots of free high quality graphics on the Internet. Here are two sites you can visit to hunt for free pictures:

▌ Yahoo's Icon page at:
http://www/yahoo.com/Computers_and_Internet/Internet/World_Wide_Web/Programming/Icons/

▌ Moby's Icon Archive at:
http://www.dsv.su.se/~matti-hu/archive.html

8.3 using html editors

If you want to simplify the process of generating web pages, there is a selection of HTML editors to choose from. These editors allow you to create HTML documents in a word-processing-like environment. They automatically produce complicated tags for graphics, frames, forms, lists, and tables. You can download most of the editors from the Net. Here is a short list:

▌ **Navigator Gold** – Visit http://home.netscape.com/

▌ **FrontPage** – Visit http://www.microsoft.com/frontpage/

▌ **Pagemill** – Visit http://www.adobe.com/prodindex/pagemill/main.html

8.4 getting your web page on the net

Once you have created your web page you need to get in on the Net. Transferring the files from your own computer onto the computer where your Internet account is located is called *uploading*. This is achieved by using an FTP utility, such as CuteFTP for Windows.

8.5 broadcasting your web page

Now that you have got you own web page you need to do some canvassing to get people to visit it. Here are a few ideas:

▌ Write to appropriate web sites and ask for a link.

▌ Get on a Mailing list and announce it.

▌ E-mail your friends and tell them about it.

▌ Use free announcing services to promote your web page. Two of the best are:

- **Promote It** at http://www.iTools.com/promote-it/
- **Submit It** at http://204.57.42.244/submit.htm

summary and conclusion

Now that you know how simple it is to create a web page, why not try creating your own and provide other health professionals/students in the world with the information you have been able to learn. It can really be a rewarding experience.

online help with your health studies and job search

"The Internet is an almost infinite library that is constantly being updated. Users can often find the facts they seek in a few minutes, without leaving their desk, and at relatively low cost." *Couchman (1999)*[18]

"The Internet is a valuable tool for accessing all kinds of information. Nurses can use the Net for their studies and need to know how to reference Internet sources." *Howe (1998)*[19]

Lecturer in Nursing
University of Wales College of Medicine,
School of Nursing Studies, Cardiff.

Universities and colleges were among the first sites to appear on the Net. Online classes are slowly appearing. Some sites are giving information about examinations, tips for success, summaries of syllabuses and so on. In this unit an attempt will be made to raise your awareness to a few interesting sites that could help you succeed on your course. Information will also be given on how to locate study tools, how to cite electronic sources and finally how to use the services on the net to find a job.

checklist

Below is a checklist of what you can expect to find out in this Unit. Read through the statements then tick (✓) the items about which you would like to know more.

I would like to find out more about:

○ **9.1 Using online tutorials to develop study skills for health courses**

○ **9.2 Evaluating health and medical resources available on the web**

○ **9.3 Referencing health material obtained from electronic sources**

○ **9.4 Finding a health or health-related job online**

Please turn over the page and read through the topics you have ticked

Learning how to learn is a skill, and a skill well worth developing. If you have just returned to full or part-time education after a long break, you will find that there is material on the Net to make you become a successful student. Take a visit to Canterbury Christ Church University College homepage at: < http://www.cant.ac.uk/study.htm >, from where you will be able to access a growing number of on-line tutorials and courseware. The page offers a comprehensive index of links to all such material.

table 9.1 **Online tutorials and courseware available at Canterbury Christ Church University College homepage**

LIST *Learning Information Skills with Technology*	**Distance Education Unit** *Department of Language Studies*
InSITE *Initiative for Staff I.T. Empowerment*	**Secondary PGCE** *Department of Education*
OLLiE *On-Line Learning Experience*	**Science Courseware** *Department of Science*
Online Tutorials *for common college pack ages*	
Examination Papers [Internal Access Only]	

The section on 'Learning Information Skills with Technology' should prove particularly useful. It is designed to enable you to collect, analyse and present your findings. The Development team who prepared that online course wrote, " . . . this course is designed to support you acquiring a range of information skills that are fundamental to success with your course of study". They also emphasise the importance of developing the skill to use NetScape effectively enough so that you can navigate around the pages in their online resource. At this web page

http://www.cant.ac.uk/cware/OLLiE/mainmenu.htm

you will find a main menu listing seven sections reproduced in Table 9.2. You should find the sections: *Self-Study Materials, Discussion Forums and WWW Resources* particularly useful.

table 9.2 **Materials available at OLLiE**

Introduction to OLLiE
A general statement about what OLLiE is
and the Course Tutors involved.

Course Outline
Using the web to display course time-
tables and course outlines. Illustrated with
some examples.

Course Evaluation
Using the web to conduct
student evaluation, monitoring
and feedback. Illustrated with
examples.

Self-Study Materials
Using the web for teaching and learning,
as well as for assessment. Illustrated
with examples.

Lecture Notes
Using the web for holding online tutorials, lecture notes
and other resources. Illustrated with examples.

Discussion Forums
Using the web for tutor/student contact,
using such methods as e-mail, newsgroups, MUDs and much more.
Illustrated with examples.

WWW Resources
A library of World Wide Web
subject-specific and teaching
and learning resources.

9.2 evaluating health and medical resources available on the web

As a student following an academic course in a college of higher education or university, you will have to write many essays. To complete these essays, you will be using, to some degree, your personal knowledge and largely information gathered from a variety of primary and secondary sources. It is important that you examine carefully the worth and arguments presented within those sources, particularly from those being published on the web. Since it is well known that anyone can publish on the Net, material from such a source is not always peer reviewed. Here are four areas that you should look at and ask yourself a few questions:

table 9.3 **Evaluating web resources**

KEY AREAS	QUESTIONS	COMMENTS
The author	What qualifies the author to speak on this subject?	Look at his qualifications, experience and possible biases as a result of his credentials.
The source	Is the publication reputable? Biased? Is it recent or out of date?	Since anyone can publish on the Net, some of the material available may not be of a high academic or professional standard. Almost anything that is more than ten years old should be treated with caution.
The arguments	What points is the author attempting to make?	Look for clarity of thoughts and supportive evidence.
The evidence	Are those points supported by reliable evidence, such as research findings?	When writing your own academic essays, you will be borrowing ideas and facts from published material. Your assignment will be valued more if the points you make are backed-up with references from reputable sources.

Being able to reference your sources clearly is an important aspect of writing academic assignments. A little time spent in understanding what is expected of you will pay dividends.

9.3.1 what is meant by referencing?

In gathering information from print sources (such as books, journals, conference papers . . .) and from electronic sources (such as CD-ROMS, the web and so on), you will use the ideas, facts, and opinions of others to support your arguments in your written assignments. On occasions you will also use the exact words that particularly support the topic you are considering in your essay. As you draw on these sources you will be expected to acknowledge the origins of the information or quotations you incorporate into your academic work. Presenting information obtained from the works of others as if it is your own is plagiarism – a habit you should avoid at all costs because it is one of the most serious academic 'crimes' you could commit in educational settings.

You will avoid plagiarism by crediting the author, whose ideas and opinions you have borrowed. References relate to a list of works cited within the text and included at the end of your written work. Two important reasons for compiling that list are:

▶ It enables readers – and markers – of your work to trace (and check) the source material.

▶ It also demonstrates that you have not just given your own opinions but have also included others opinions to illustrate a point or offer support for an argument.

9.3.2 formats of references

In preparing your written work, you should use the style of referencing specified by your institution. If you are not sure which one to use, check with your course tutor. The Harvard and the Vancouver styles continue to be the two most commonly used systems for referencing printed materials within books and periodicals. Here is a quick reminder of those two styles of referencing as they are applied to printed materials.

▶ **Harvard system**: This system is often referred to as the 'author/date' system (Dwyer, 1995),[20] and is used mainly in nursing and the social sciences (St. George's Library, 1999).[21] When using this system, if the author's name occurs naturally in the sentence, references are cited in the main body of the text like this: Chellen (1995) wrote about the . . . ; otherwise like this: (Chellen, 1995) at the end of the sentence. This is then listed alphabetically by surname in a reference list at the end of the work. This **reference list** follows a general form as illustrated in Table 9.4.

▶ **Vancouver system**: This system is also referred to as the 'numerical system' (Dwyer, 1995). When using this system – which most academic/medical journals prefer – references are numbered consecutively in the text and are listed in numerical order at the end of the essay/paper. The *reference list* follows the general form as illustrated in Table 9.4.

Information on electronic sources can be classified under two broad headings: 'Internet Sources' and 'Non-Internet Sources'. The first category includes material from Electronic journals, Individual works on web sites, Personal e-mail, Mailing lists, Newsgroups, FTP sites, Gopher sites, and online databases. The second category includes material from electronic media like CD-ROMS and Computer disks.

Unfortunately, as yet there is no agreed and fixed standard for referencing Internet publications. One particular problem is the temporary nature of much of the material made available on the Internet. This makes it hard for the scientific community to decide whether it can accept the validity of a non-permanent document as a legitimate reference source. Indeed, writers like McKenzie (1996, p55)[16] have rightly argued that only archived, retrievable versions may be regarded as valid. But, as electronic sources become an intrinsic part of your scholarly interaction, it is essential when referencing these sources that you do so with the same degree of care as for printed material.

table 9.4 **Citation systems for for books and periodicals**

	HARVARD STYLE	VANCOUVER STYLE
BOOKS	Author(s)/editor surname, initials. (Year of publication) <u>Title of book</u>, Edition [if later than first]. Place/Town of publication: Publisher's name.	(No.) Author/s, Initials Title. (Edition). City: Publisher, Year: (Page numbers)
	Example: Chellen, S. S. & Chellen, P. D. (1995) <u>Word for Windows for the Caring Professions – A Beginner's Workbook</u>. London: Cassell plc.	**Example:** (1) Chellen, S.S., & Chellen, P. D. *Word for Windows for the Caring Professions – A Beginner's Workbook*. London: Cassell plc. 1995.
ARTICLES	Author(s) surname, initials (Year of publication) Article title. *Journal title. Volume number* (issue number) Date of issue: first and last pages.	(No.) Author/s. Title {Type of article}. *Journal*, Year, Month; *Volume* (Issue): Page numbers.
	Example: Chellen, S. S. (1995) A Layman's Guide to IT, In *Occupational Health – a Journal for Healthworkers*, 47(10), Oct 10:pp 351–2 & 354–5.	**Example:** (2) Chellen, S.S. A Layman's Guide to IT, In *Occupational Health – a Journal for Healthworkers*, 1995. Oct 10; 47(10): 351–2 & 354–5.

For more information on Harvard style visit:
< http://www.cant.ac.uk/depts/services/library/harvard.htm >
< http://www.sghms.ac.uk/library/harefern.htm >

To assist you, various writers have suggested ways of adapting the Harvard and Vancouver systems to apply them to electronic sources. Below is my adaptation of the two systems, offered as a guide only. You should also consult the course handbook in your institution. To allow your source to be checked and verified, you should cite the reference in the text in the same way as you would for printed materials, and then use the format indicated in Table 9.6 to list the references making sure to include all the information given in Table 9.5.[22]

table 9.5 **Essential Information required in reference citations**

BIBLIOGRAPHICAL DETAILS	COMMENTS
Author: The name(s) of the person(s) or publishing body responsible for the document.	This is usually the first element of a citation. If the author is not available, the title becomes the first element of the reference, and the work is alphabetised in the reference list by the first significant word in the title.
Date: The year, month and day when the electronic form of the publication was created or updated and/or accessed.	This validates the existence of a cited file at a given time, and indirectly indicates the possible version of, say, a database when this becomes difficult to determine. The access date element is always the last element of a citation and enclosed in square brackets. This allows for later modification or removal of information.
Title: This is the main heading on the electronic document being cited or in the Titlebar ie, the blue strip at the top of the screen.	If later than the first, this should include an edition or version number.
Medium: ie, type of resource the information is stored on, eg, online, CD-ROM, Laserdisk, Videodisk, Diskette, e-mail, WWW etc.	This is to show that the reference source is not a printed book or article. In situations where it is difficult to detect the medium, for example when using a database on a college computer network, then use the generic term "electronic" to distinguish the cited electronic references from print ones.
Location: wherever the user has to go to in order to find the document in question, eg, http, ftp address, etc.	The golden rule here is accuracy. Be extra careful with spelling and punctuation.
Commands	Any other instructions needed to locate the document (if relevant).

9.3.3 referencing internet sources

table 9.6a **World Wide Web and electronic journals**

	HARVARD STYLE	VANCOUVER STYLE
	Author(s), initials. (Date created/ updated). Document Title. [Medium]. Location. [Date accessed]	(No.) Author(s), initials. Document Title. [Medium]. Year. Location. [Date accessed].
Example 1	ENB Report On Practice Placement Review Visits – Learning Disability Nursing MAY 1997 – APRIL 1998. [WWW]. Available from: < http://www.enb.org.uk/ldplace.htm > [Accessed: 1998, November 27]	(1) ENB Report On Practice Placement Review Visits – Learning Disability Nursing MAY 1997 – APRIL 1998. [WWW]. Available from: < http://www.enb.org.uk/ldplace.htm > [Accessed: 12 January 1999].
Example 2	Allen, M. (no date). SPSS for Windows Version 7 – A review. In *On-line Journal of Nursing Informatics* 1(1). [WWW]. Available from: < http://cac.psu.edu/~dxm12/spss.html > [Accessed: 1999, January 15]	(1) Allen, M. SPSS for Windows Version 7 – A review in *On-line Journal of Nursing Informatics* 1(1). [WWW]. Available from: < http://cac.psu.edu/~dxm12/spss.html > [Accessed: 15 January 1998].
Comments		

▷ *Often the author's name, or a link to the author's homepage, can be found at the bottom of the web page. In some cases, the author may be the organisation responsible for the site.*

▷ *Many WWW pages now include the date when it was last updated, which is equivalent to the publication date. If not, make sure you include the date you accessed the page.*

▷ *The title of a web page will normally be the main heading on the page, or in the Titlebar – ie, the blue strip at the top of the screen.*

▷ *When including URL it is best to use angle brackets (< >) around the URL to set it off. Without such delimiters, inexperienced readers may misinterpret following punctuation as part of the URL (even though URLs shouldn't end in periods, commas, or semicolons). Also only move to a new line following a forward slash(/).*

▷ *Use a name, not a number, for the host part of the URL — for example, http://www.eeicom.com/eye/, not http://204.7.7.4/eye/.*

▷ *Remember URLs are case sensitive ie, they recognise the difference between upper and lower case. Make sure they are given accurately.*

▷ *Some web pages are part of a larger set of documents, such as an electronic journal or book; for them it may be appropriate to include the title of the larger publication.*

table 9.6b **Online databases**

	HARVARD STYLE	VANCOUVER STYLE
	Author(s), initials (Date created/ updated). Document title. [Medium]. Online database name on host. Search command. [Accessed date].	(No.) Author(s), initials. Document Title. Year. [Medium]. Online database name on host. Search command. [Date accessed].
Example 1	Cort. E. (no date) Nurses' attitudes to sexuality in caring for cancer patients. In *Nursing Times*, 21 Oct. 1998, 94(42):pp54–56. [Online ENB Healthcare Database]. Available from: < http://www.enb.org.uk/cgi-bin/hcdsearch >. In Search box type: CANCER PATIENTS [Accessed: 2 February 1999].	(1) Cort. E. "Nurses' attitudes to sexuality in caring for cancer patients". In *Nursing Times*, 21 Oct. 1998, 94(42): pp54-56. [Online ENB Healthcare Database]. Available from: < http://www.enb.org.uk/cgi-bin/hcd search >. In Search box type: CANCER PATIENTS. [Accessed: 2 February 1999].
Example 2	Chellen, S.S. (1982) A Layman's guide to IT. In *Occupational Health: A Journal for Occupational Health Nurses* 47(10):pp351–2, 354–5. [Online Database: CINAHL]. Available from Electronic Services – BIOMED: < http://biomed.niss.ac.uk > Select Author then type: Chellen. [Accessed: 5 February 1999].	(2) Chellen, S.S. "A Layman's guide to IT". In *Occupational Health: A Journal for Occupational Health Nurses* 47(10):pp351–2, 354–5. 1982. [Online Database: CINAHL]. Available from Electronic Services – BIOMED: < http://biomed.niss.ac.uk > Select Author then type: Chellen. [Accessed: 5 February 1999].
Comments	▌ To facilitate location of the article, it is extremely important to include the keyword or keyphrase you used to access the article in the database.	

table 9.6c **FTP sites**

	HARVARD STYLE	VANCOUVER STYLE
	Author(s), initials. (Date created/ updated). Title of document or file. Edition/Version [Medium]. Location. [Date accessed].	(No.) Author(s), initials Title of document or file. Edition/Version. [Medium]. Year. Location. [Date accessed].
Example	RANKIN, B (1997, Jan 27). Accessing the Internet by e-mail, (6th Ed.). [FTP]. Available from: < ftp://ftp.mailbase.ac.uk/pub/lists/lis-iis/files/e-access-inet.txt > [Accessed: Y, M D].	(1) RANKIN, B Accessing the Internet by e-mail, (6th Ed.). [FTP]. 1997. Available from: < ftp://ftp.mailbase.ac.uk/pub/lists/ lis-iis/files/e-access-inet.txt > [Accessed: D M Y].
Comments	▌ When including URL use angle brackets (< >) around the URL to set it off and only move to a new line following a forward slash (/). ▌ Use a name, not a number, for the host part of the URL.	

table 9.6d **Gopher sites**

	HARVARD STYLE	VANCOUVER STYLE
Gopher	Author(s), initials (Date created/ updated). Document Title. Version/ Format. [Medium]. Location. [Date accessed].	(No.) Author(s), initials Document Title. [Medium]. Year. Location. [Date accessed] .
Example	MIT Center for Space Research (1997, Jan. 20) Space Shuttle News. [Gopher]. Available from: < Gopher://gopher.umds.ac.uk:70/00 technical/space-shuttle-news > [Accessed: Y, M D].	(1) MIT Center for Space Research Space Shuttle News. [Gopher]. 1997. Available from: < Gopher://gopher.umds.ac.uk: 70/ 00/technical/space-shuttle-news > [Accessed: D M Y].
Comments	▶ *Refer to Table 9.6c.*	

table 9.6e **Personal e-mail messages (archived works)**

	HARVARD STYLE	VANCOUVER STYLE
	Author(s), initials (date posted). Subject line from posting. [Medium]. Location. [Date accessed].	(No.) Author(s), initials Subject line from posting. [Medium]. Date Posted. Location. [Date accessed].
Example	RIUS-RIU, M (1998, May 22) Copyright on the Internet [Personal e-mail to Chellen. SS]. Available from: < ssc1@cant.ac.uk >] [Accessed: 1998, May 23].	(1) RIUS-RIU, M. Copyright on the Internet [Personal e-mail to Chellen. S.S.]. 22 May 1998. Available from:< ssc1@cant.ac.uk > [Accessed: 23 May 1998].
Comments	▶ *When including Address use angle brackets (< >) around the address to set it off.* ▶ *If your source is controversial or temporary then keep a hard copy, just in case you are requested to produce it. Better still attach a hard copy to your essay, thesis etc.* ▶ *Personal e-mail should be treated in a similar manner to other non-electronic forms of personal communication. It is essential to request permission from the author before quoting an e-mail message in essays, especially if you are including the author's e-mail address, otherwise, as [Steve Gilligan (see p. 109)] points out, you may break both Copyright and Data Protection regulations.*	

table 9.6f **E-mail messages from usenet newsgroups**

	HARVARD STYLE	VANCOUVER STYLE
	Author(s), initials (Date posted). Subject line from posting in newsgroups. [Medium]. Newsgroup name.	(No.) Author(s), initials. Subject line from posting in newsgroups. Date posted. [Medium]. Newsgroup name.
Example	Strong, A. (1998, December 26) Clinical Assistant: A new nursing role? [Usenet]. Available from: < uk.sci.med.nursing >.	(1) STRONG, A. Clinical Assistant: A new nursing role? 26 December 1998. [Usenet]. Available from: < uk.sci.med.nursing >.
Comments	▶ *Use posting date, to allow tracing of message through archives.* ▶ *The title is the subject line/header.*	

table 9.6g **E-mail message from mailing lists**

	HARVARD STYLE	VANCOUVER STYLE
	Author(s), initials (Date posted). Subject line from posting on listname. [Medium]. Server host address.	(No.) Author(s), initials Document Title. Date posted. [Medium]. Server host address.
Example	MACLEOD, R. (1996, January 19). Internet resources Newsletter – latest issue on LIS-LINK. [Mailing Lists]. Available from: < mailbase@mailbase.ac.uk >	(1) MACLEOD, R. Internet resources Newsletter – latest issue on LIS-LINK. 19 Jan. 1996. [Mailing Lists]. Available from: < mailbase@mailbase.ac.uk >
Comments	▶ *The title is the subject line.* ▶ *By using posting date, it allows tracing of the message through archives. However, such messages although archived are often kept for a short time. Consequently, some institutions may not consider this source as suitable for referencing.*	

9.3.4 referencing non-internet sources

table 9.6h **Computer disks**

	HARVARD STYLE	VANCOUVER STYLE
	Author(s), initials (Date created/ updated). Document title. Version. [Medium]. Town: Publisher.	(No.) Author(s), initials Document title. Version. Date created/updated. [Medium]. Town: Publisher.
Example	Education and Training Programme in IM & T for Clinicians (1996, Sept.) Champion Database. Version 3.2. [Disk]. Bristol: Blackwell Idealist.	(1) Education and Training Programme in IM & T for Clinicians Champion Database. Version 3.2. September 1996. [Disk]. Bristol: Blackwell Idealist.

table 9.6i **CD-ROM databases**

	HARVARD STYLE	VANCOUVER STYLE
	Author(s), initials (Date created/ updated). Document title. Version. [Medium]. Town: Publisher.	(No.) Author(s), initials Document title. Version. Date created/updated. [Medium]. Town: Publisher.
Example	Caredata CD: the social and community care database. [CD-ROM]. 1997, April. London: National Institute for Social Work.	(1) Caredata CD: the social and community care database. [CD-ROM]. April 1997. London: National Institute for Social Work.

table 9.6j **CD-ROM texts**

	HARVARD STYLE	VANCOUVER STYLE
	Author(s), initials (Date created/ updated). Document title. Version. [Medium]. Town: Publisher.	(No.) Author(s), initials Document title. Version. Date created/updated. [Medium]. Town: Publisher.
Example 1	Using Technology to find Clinical Information. [CD-ROM]. 1998, April. Bristol: Enabling People Team NHS Executive – South & West. Tel 0117 984 1904.	(1) NHS Executive Using Technology to find Clinical Information. [CD-ROM]. April,1998. Bristol: Enabling People Team NHS Executive – South & West. Tel 0117 984 1904.
Example 2	Using IM & T in Clinical Practice. [CD-ROM]. 1998, April. Bristol: Enabling People Team NHS Executive – South & West. Tel 0117 984 1904.	(2) Using IM & T in Clinical Practice. [CD-ROM]. April,1998. Bristol: Enabling People Team NHS Executive – South & West. Tel 0117 984 1904.
Example 3	Mathers, L.H., Chase, R.A., & Dev, P.A. (1996, Oct.). Clinical Anatomy Interactive Lesson. [CD-ROM]. St Louis: Mosby.	(3) Mathers, L.H., Chase, R.A., & Dev, P.A. Clinical Anatomy Interactive Lesson. Oct., 1996. [CD-ROM]. St Louis: Mosby.
Comments	*In examples 1 and 2 above, the title is the first element of the reference. In the reference list for the Harvard style, the work is alphabetised using the first significant word in the title.*	

9.4 finding a health or health-related job online

After all your hard work and successful completion of your course, you quite rightly would like to be rewarded with a suitable job. This can be a very trying time. Once again you will find the Net coming to your rescue.

▌ Take a visit to the following UK sites where you will find thousands of vacancies.

▌ The PeopleBank (Fig.9.1) at http://www.peoplebank.com Here as a jobseeker you won't have to pay anything. Simply fill in the online registration form, and submit your CV or browse through the database of job vacancies.

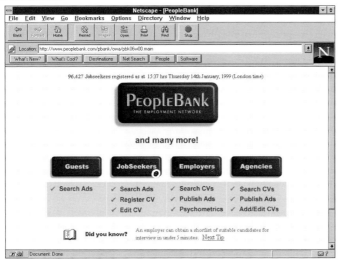

◁ fig. 9.1 **The PeopleBank homepage**

▶ WorkWeb at http://www.workweb.co.uk. Here you will find searchable job categories, support and additional information. You simply pick a category and search the database. See Fig 9.2.

▶ You can also scan professional journals online. Go to http://www.yahoo.co.uk/Reference/journals. Select the 'health' category and choose a journal to read online.

▶ Subscribe to newsgroups, and filter the newsgroup list. Useful ones are alt.jobs; **alt.jobs.overseas**; **uk.jobs**; **sci.med.jobs**.

▶ If you subscribe to Mailing list, you might be pleasantly surprised to see job vacancies being automatically delivered to your mailbox.

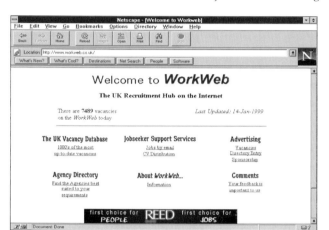

◁ fig. 9.2 **Looking for a job on the WorkWeb site**

◁ **Step 1**
Point and click on the category labelled **The UK Vacancy Database** and you will be taken to the next screen shown below.

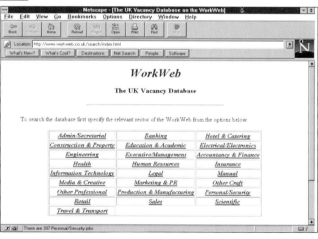

Step 2 ▷
Point and click on the category labelled **Health** and you will be taken to the next screen shown below.

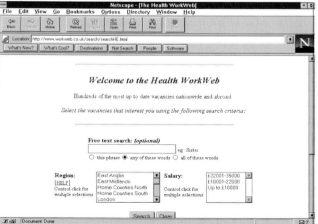

◁ **Step 3**
Now simply follow the onscreen instructions.

summary and conclusion

Online tutorials can provide a valuable way of developing your skills in learning. By all means use the health information on the Net to help in your assignments, but do take care with this, as the information may not be reliable. Be extra careful when referencing sources from the Net.

question 1

what is a PDF document?

NOTE

Normally a PDF document has the extension .pdf. In Windows (or on the Macintosh) you can also open a PDF document by double-clicking the file icon. If double-clicking a file on the Macintosh platform does not open the file in your Acrobat Viewer, use File | Open to open the file, then close the file, and try again.

answer: Documents can be saved to disks in a variety of formats. When accessing online journals, such as Nursing Standard Online, you will find that some documents have been prepared in a special format called Adobe PDF, which stands for "Portable Document Format". To view, navigate, and print such documents, you need a special program called Acrobat Reader. You should find this program on the desktop of your college computer network. Adobe Acrobat Reader is usually available free of charge. Your college computing department should be able to give you a copy to use on your home system. If not, you can always visit the Adobe website http://cep.lse.ac.uk/pdf.html and download yourself a free copy.

When you come across a PDF document, you will first have to save it to disk using a unique filename. Then to read it, do the following:

▶ Activate the Acrobat Reader program.

▶ Choose **File** from the menubar.

▶ Choose the command **Open**.

▶ In the **Open File** dialogue box, highlight the filename, and click on the command **Open**. *The article you saved should open into the Acrobat Viewer window.*

question 2

what are cookies?

answer: Cookies are small text files that are stored on your computer's hard disk when you visit certain web sites. They serve a variety of purposes to the author of a web site and can be of some benefit to those who visit the site. For example, when you have visited a web site and accepted a Cookie, a unique code that identifies you is saved to your hard disk. An advantage of having accepted a Cookie is that when you revisit the site, you may not be required to go through the process of supplying your name and password. You may even be allowed to access restricted areas of a site. Web creators (particularly those who rely on advertisements for their income) often use Cookies to keep a log of the paths you follow through the site and the pages you decided to visit. This helps them to know a bit more about your interests, and enables them to target you with the kind of adverts most likely to capture your attention. When you visit certain web sites for the first time, a dialogue box will appear offering you a Cookie. You have the choice of accepting or rejecting the offer by clicking on the appropriate option. Cookies are quite safe. Contrary to popular belief, they can't be used to spy on you ie, read any other data from your hard disk or find out what software you have installed.

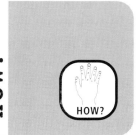

How does Cookie work?

Cookies work in the following way: When you are surfing the web pages and follow a link to re-visit a web site, your browser sends the Cookie containing the URL of the site as you click the hyperlink. This immediately informs the site that you have been there before. You may receive a nice personalised welcome, such as "Hello Syd, this is your 3rd visit".

Although Cookies are quite harmless, you may object to the fact that others are attempting to use your hard disk to store those small text files. Fortunately, you can set your browser to warn you when a site is attempting to store a Cookie on your hard disk. A dialogue box like the one shown below should appear:

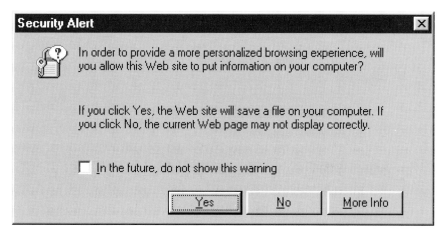

Sadly, when you decide to reject a Cookie you may find that some sites will not let you in. A smarter way of dealing with Cookies is to accept them and then delete them when you have finished surfing.

To locate and view Cookies

▶ Open your Windows directory folder, and then. . .

▶ Open the Cookies directory folder.

▶ Point and double-click on a Cookie header to open its contents into a window for reading.

To delete a Cookie

▶ Point to the Cookie header and click the RIGHT mouse button to open the submenu.

▶ Click on the Delete command on the submenu to get off that Cookie.

what are computer viruses and are they harmful?

An <u>operating</u> <u>system</u> is a complex computer program used to control, assist or supervise all other programs that run on a computer system.

answer: There will be occasions when you will be using your college computer network to download information from the Net to take home to use on your computer system. Similarly there may be times when you may start preparing your assignment on your home system and then decide to finish it off on the college computer network or vice versa. The risk of exporting or importing a virus is real. So what is a computer virus? It is a category of software which infects other software programs and data files, and which replicates itself. A virus can spread via disks and the main problem is usually its side-effects. Viruses have been known to transmit themselves over an entire network. There are over 200 viruses at large and the number is steadily growing. 95% of viruses simply replicate themselves, cause your keyboard to beep every time you hit a key on your keyboard on a particular day of the month, or display a message on your computer screen. However, a minute few can be problematic. The most serious type is the one that infects an **Operating System** as this governs the whole running of a computer system. Fortunately, there are vaccine programs that can deal with viruses. Although virus infections can be regarded as just another PC problem, the more preventive measures you can take against viruses entering a system the better, since getting rid of a virus can take time, and time is money. Table Q1 outlines ways of minimising the risk. For additional information pay a visit to Dr Solomon's web site:

http://www.drsolomon.co.uk/home/home.cfm

table Q1 **How to protect your computer system against viruses**

Software	Use only software that comes from reputable sources. Avoid using pirated versions of software
Compartmentalisation	Keep program files and data files in separate directories or better still on separate disks.
Vaccine	Inoculate your computer against known viruses
Virus guard	Install a virus guard on your computer.
Backups	Maintain regular backups of all your files
Screening	Ensure that any disk you receive or bring home with data is virus-free by checking it using the latest version of a virus-checking program like Dr Solomon.
Performance	You should investigate and rectify any flaws in a widely used program as soon as they come to light.
Access control	Prevent unauthorised access to your data files or programs by using access controls such as passwords.

what are plug-ins?

answer: Web pages are getting smarter and smarter. Web site creators are increasingly making imaginative use of multimedia facilities. However, your browser may not be able to support these novelties. Plug-ins are software programs that extend the capabilities of your web browser in a certain way, such as allowing you to hear live audio broadcasts or view video movies. A plug-in is installed on your hard disk using the instructions that come with the plug-in. After installation your NetScape browser uses the plug-in's capabilities like other built-in NetScape features. There are literally hundreds of plug-ins out there to enable you to access different types of multimedia file. For example, you may visit a web site that uses RealAudio plug-ins for music, speech, or a mixture of the two. RealAudio will allow you to hear musical sound while a file is being downloaded. If you are using Internet Explorer, the RealAudio plug-in is bundled with it. However, if you are using NetScape or any other browser, you can download the player software from this web site:

< http://www.realaudio.com >

. . . and install it on your computer. Another useful plug-in is: **Adobe's Acrobat Reader** – a PDF (portable document format) reader that enables you to view elaborate electronic documents stored in PDF format.

(< http://www.adobe.com/products/acrobat/readstep.html >).

what is a cache and how does it work?

answer: When logging on to NetScape on your college network to surf the Net, you might see a dialogue box with a message asking if you want the system to maximise your cache. I suggest you click on the YES button. Cache temporarily stores the information on a page in your computer. The first time you ask for a page, your browser retrieves the page from the network. No pages are permanently stored in a cache. If you request a page you have seen before, your browser checks to see if the page is available in a cache. For example, if you use the BACK button on your browser to display a page, a cache can display the page more quickly than the network can retransmit it.

what should I know about firewalls?

answer: Data security and privacy is extremely important in healthcare. Using a firewall it is possible to protect one or more computers with Internet connections from access by external computers connected to the Internet. A firewall is a network configuration, created by software and hardware, that forms a boundary between networked computers within the firewall from those outside the firewall. The computers within the firewall become a secure subset with internal access capabilities and shared resources not available to the computers on the outside. A firewall is commonly used to protect information such as data files within an organisation site. A firewall reduces the risk of intrusion by unauthorised people from the Internet. However, the same security measures can limit or require special software for those inside the firewalls who wish to access information on the outside.

question 7

should anyone give out a credit card number on the internet?

answer: At some point on your course you will need to buy books. While busy surfing, you may arrive at an Internet bookshop where you decide to order a book but wonder whether it is safe to make the payment using your credit card. Stop for a moment and consider how you use your credit or debit card in the 'real world'. For example, do you always ask for the carbon paper after signing for a credit card purchase? The truth is, card numbers are so easy to steal. Stealing credit card numbers over the Net is much harder, because it takes a lot of effort and technical know-how. One credit number is unlikely to warrant the effort. Nevertheless, to make the hacker's job even more difficult, most web sites at which you can use your credit card run on secure servers. Furthermore, NetScape allows you to enter your credit card number on a secure (https) NetScape Navigator form for it to be transmitted over the Internet to a secure server without the risk of an intermediary obtaining your credit card information. The NetScape clearly states that "the security features offered by NetScape Communications technology prevent fraud that could otherwise occur as information passes through Internet computers".

WARNING!

However, before you enter into any commercial transaction over the Net, be sure you are willing to trust the server administrator with your credit card number in the same way as you would if you were telling someone your credit card number over the telephone.

question 8

what is home highway and how does it work?

answer: Whilst your standard phone line uses analogue technology, Home Highway – a new service from BT – uses digital *ISDN2e* technology to give you flexibility and speed. Home Highway upgrades your existing standard telephone line by transforming it into two lines, each of which can be used for analogue and digital access simultaneously. The digital signal is far clearer than an analogue signal, allowing for greatly improved performance when using a computer. According to BT (1998)[23] "[with Home Highway] digital computer access is over four times faster than an analogue modem operating at 28.8K and can usually connect in a few seconds compared to the 45 seconds it can take using an analogue modem". With Home Highway, you have access to unique multi-tasking opportunities at an increased speed, such as:

▶ A blistering 128K speed when browsing the Internet and downloading stuff.

▶ A 64K speed on one line whilst making and receiving phone calls on the other.

▶ A 64K speed when using two PCs to work on the Internet at the same time.

▶ The flexibility of 64K speed for surfing the Net with your PC while simultaneously using your phone for making and receiving calls or faxes.

For more Information on Home Highway, such as equipment, installation, charges and other Q&A, pay a visit to the BT homepage at:

< http:///www.homehighway.bt.com >

. . . or call a BT adviser on Freefone *0800 222 444.*

question 9

what are trolls?

answer: A troll is a posting deliberately intended to provoke a flame war on Newsgroups. The term "troll" has its root in fishing: "trolling" is casting a bait a long way out and pulling it slowly back in order to attract the fish to your boat. In a similar way, gather a collection of newcomers to newsgroups and then slowly taken to tasks. Here is an example of a troll:

It is well known that the 'H' in 'Margaret H. Thatcher' stands for "Hilda". Now, if someone comes along who insists until he is blue in the face that it stands for "Hilary" you'd want to put him right, right? Wrong. That's what he wants. If you dare get involved, you will be rushing to the bait.

question 10

what is spamming?

answer: This is a net expression for sending the same message to multiple *newsgroups* or *e-mail* recipients regardless of their interest (or lack of it). Most 'spamming' consist of unsolicited advertisements. Apart from the personal aggravation it causes, spamming is also a massive waste of _bandwidth_. Hoyler (1997)[2] relates an interesting case of spamming that ought to serve as a warning to all of us:

'Cantor and Seigal was a firm of US lawyers who went in for one of the less nice legal scams in recent years. It's not very well-known that the United States runs a Green Card lottery every year. Anyone can go along to the US embassy, fill in *a card with their name and address, and every year or so they make a draw and the few people whose cards are drawn (from the thousands submitted) are given a Green Card – that is, full US citizenship. In the last few years, some firms of lawyers have exploited this by offering their services to "help you get US citizenship" – that is, they will charge you £100 to fill in a card for you and put it in on your behalf. You sometimes see adverts for these services in the small ads in the back of newspapers. Cantor and Seigal took this to extremes, by putting out their advert on the Internet. In particular, they sent a copy to every single newsgroup'.*

This act is regarded as spamming and it is frowned on. Now, there are two possible ways of dealing with this sort of behaviour. Firstly, you can put a complaint to their Internet Service Provider or System Administrator. Secondly, you can use a technique called "mail bombing" ie, you send an e-mail containing a very large meaningless attachment-file to the perpetrators of the spam. If the volume is large enough it will cause the Internet Service Provider's system to crash. According to Hoyler (1997),[3] this is exactly what happened to Cantor and Siegal. A large volume of abusive e-mail was sent to Cantor and Seigal putting their Internet Service Provider's system out of action for several days. Cantor and Seigal's account was cancelled and they were sued for damages by their Service Provider.

So there you have it!

question 11

what are cyber cafés?

answer: In the last couple of years, a few cafés and pubs, besides offering tea, coffee, beer and so on, have started making available to their clients computers with Internet access. Users are charged a fee per hour to use the computers to access the Internet, and very often it is necessary for one to book time in advance (especially at lunch times, evenings and weekends).
Here is a selective list of UK Cyber Cafés:

- 3W Café at 4, Market Place, Bracknell, Berkshire;

- Cyberia Café at 39 Whitfield Street, London;

- Electric Frog at 42-44 Cockburn Street, Edinburgh;

- Planet 13 at 25 High Cross Street, St. Austell, Cornwall;

- Revelations at Shaftesbury Square, Belfast;

- The Edge at St George's Centre, St Ann's Road, Harrow, Middlesex;

- Punters Cyber Café at 111 Arundel Street, Sheffield;

- CyberZone at 1 Dingwall Road, Croydon, Surrey;

- Chaucer Cyberspace at Chaucer Tech. School, Spring Lane, Canterbury, Kent.

How to find more answers to questions?

There are several websites that have a section called FAQ (Frequently Asked Questions). Here are two web sites that will give you answers to many questions you may care to ask:

- http://www.columbia.edu./cu/healthwise/alice.html

- http://www.patents.com/weblaw.sht

HOW?

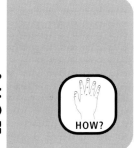

question **12**

answer: Copyright law usually gives the owner the exclusive right to control copying of a writing, recording, picture, or electronic transcription. When it comes to Cyberspace, the law is frustratingly vague and difficult to interpret. But to avoid copyright infringement here are a few points that Net surfers should keep in mind:

what about copyright law and the net?

- Almost everything you produce yourself on the Net is protected under copyright law. As soon you have written your work eg, e-mail message, posting to newsgroups, or a web creation – it's automatically copyrighted (without the need to send it anywhere, or even put a copyright notice on it). However, having a copyright symbol on your page leaves no one in any doubt.

- Copyright law does not mean that you cannot use another's work for inspiration, but simply that you are not allowed to copy it without permission. Do remember though, ideas, facts, titles, names, or short phrases are not copyrighted.

- A message to a newsgroup is under copyright, but as it was posted onto a discussion list, the writer gave an implicit licence for others to quote the person in their response.

- Linking one's homepage to someone else's is becoming a common practice. There does not appear to be a problem in this area as long as you do not try to take credit for the other person's work. By being on the web, there is an implied permission for others to add a link. You are not legally required to inform the web site that you are adding to his/her homepage, although this would be good netiquette. However, it is not permissible to use someone's actual list of links if that list demonstrates some originality.

- Provided images and graphics on the web are in the **Public Domain**, it is legal to use them. Otherwise, you must obtain permission from the copyright holder.

- There is a lot of excellent material on the Internet that is Public Domain and free for anyone to copy and use. However, unless the right to copy is implicit or the author has made it explicitly free to copy ("you are free to

> **Public Domain** is material that, for whatever reason, is not protected by copyright law and can be used freely without permission. An example is a copyright that has expired.
>
> **TECHNO TALK**

use this material"), you will be wise to keep your hands off. (The law here is somewhat fuzzy.)

Finally the law in Cyberspace is continuously evolving. To help you keep yourself up-to-date here are four web sites:

- **10 Big Myths About Copyright Explained**
  http://www.clari.net/brad/copymyths.html

- **Web Law FAQ**
  http://www.patents.com/weblaw.sht

- **Cyberspace Law for Non-lawyers**
  http://www.lawnewsnetwork.com

- **The Copyright Website**
  http://www.benedict.com/)

appendix 1 the user agreement

Here is a typical User agreement that you can expect from colleges or universities when you register to use computing facilities. Following registration, you are given an account ie, a username and password. Acceptance of this account implies that you implicitly agree to comply with the College regulations governing the use of computing facilities. The full text of these "Regulations for the use of the Computing Service" may be issued to you and/or may be displayed in computing laboratories and in other places eg, students' notice board. It is your responsibility to read these Regulations and to ensure that you comply with them, as any breach will render you liable to disciplinary action. Here is a summary:

 These rules apply to anyone using any kind of computer hardware or software at the College, for any purpose, even if it is their own equipment and even if it is only connected to the College through a network or telephone line. They also apply to anyone here using the computer facilities of another University or College.

 You are required to register, or be registered, in order to use College computing facilities. Any user identification or password you are given is for you alone: do not tell anyone your registration details and do not attempt to use anyone else's. If you leave the College or change your course you must tell User Services.

 Special permission is needed to use computers for personal, commercial or outside work use. There may be charges for some types of computer use.

 You must ensure that you know how to use the equipment. Follow the instructions for starting and finishing sessions and while you are using computing equipment.

 You must not damage, interfere with, or change any hardware or software; if you do you will be charged with the cost of putting it right. You need permission to move anything or to connect any new hardware. Only use authorised software. You may not load new software without permission. Do not introduce, or risk introducing, computer viruses or anything similar. Do not interfere with other users or their data or software.

 You must not create, bring in, display, produce or circulate any offensive material.

- Smoking, eating and drinking near computing equipment may cause damage and is not allowed.

- Old data and uncollected printouts may be removed by housekeeping procedures. Do not rely on them being retained for you.

- The College does not accept responsibility for any loss caused by your use of computing facilities.

- Any breach of these Regulations may also constitute a breach of criminal or civil law but will certainly render you liable to disciplinary action.

Reproduced by kind permission of Computing Services,
Canterbury Christ Church University College.

appendix 2   service providers
2.1 uk online services

Here is a selected list of the online services available with a brief discussion of the first four. You will find a comprehensive list in *Internet* magazine. All the companies on the list will provide you (on request) with free software to subscribe. Do not forget to ask them for details of subscription schemes on offer and do read the small print. Read Section 2.3.5 if you have not already done so. It is also recommended that you browse each service before committing yourself.

NOTE

Information about service providers is subject to change. Details given here are for guidance only and were accurate at time of compilation. Inclusion does not imply endorsement.

COMPANY	TELEPHONE	E-MAIL ADDRESS	WEB SITE ADDRESS
CompuServe	0800 289378	70006.101@compserve.com	http://www.compserve.com
America Online (AOL)	0800 279 1234	queryuk@aol.com	http://www.aol.com
Microsoft Network (MSN)	0345 002000		http://www.msn.com
Virgin Net	0500 558800		http://www.virgin.net
Delphi	0171-757 7080	ukservice@delphi.com	http://www.delphi.co.uk
CIX	0181 296 9666	Sales@compulink.co.uk	http://www.compulink.co.uk
ClaraNet	0171-647 1000	Sales@clara.net	http://www.clara.net

2.1.1 compuserve

CompuServe (or CIS, an acronym for CompuServe Information Service) covers several subjects including interactive chat rooms. When you sign on, opening screens provide labels or icons for broad categories, such as news, entertainment, computers, health, and so on. Click on any one of these and you will find a subcategory of choices. Many retail companies have their own forums offering advice and product support. The program used to move around is fairly smart but not quite as easy as, say, America Online. It is also somewhat slow in use. The UK specific content is sparse, though the company is trying hard to improve this. CompuServe charges by service categories: most things are included in a basic monthly fee with an additional surcharge for some "premium services". Over 3,000 products and services (eg, news, weather, entertainments, health, etc) are available to members for up to five hours a month with additional hourly charge for extra time. Premium services (eg, many of the online databases), unfortunately carry surcharges that vary from service to service – rates are available online. For additional information visit: http://www.compuserve.co.uk

2.1.2 america online

America Online (AOL) is very user-friendly and is therefore a good choice for inexperienced computer-users. It has the simplest pricing plan. You pay a flat rate fee for five hours of use and a nominal hourly rate for every hour after the initial five. This includes every service you can find on AOL, except a handful of special services such as sending paper ("snail") mail or faxes through AOL. The content provided is quite similar to that of CompuServe, though there is plenty of UK content. One major benefit is that it allows you to have five different e-mail addresses.

2.1.3 the microsoft network (msm)

MSM has a stylish, modern appearance, but requires Windows 95 or later in order to run. Your computer, too, has to have a reasonably fast processor (100Mhz or above). Access to a standard array of subjects is essentially the same as AOL and CompuServe. It has a US bias and is geared more towards entertainment than information.

2.1.4 virgin net

This is relatively new on the scene. It is a UK-only company; hence the content that is included is UK-specific, with news, sport, chat rooms, and hundreds of ready-sorted links to places of interest on the Internet.

2.2 uk internet service providers

Here is a selected list of ISPs. All ISPs listed below offer basic services of e-mail, www, FTP, Telnet, Gopher, IRC and newsgroups access. See column 5 for additional details.

COMPANY	TELEPHONE	E-MAIL ADDRESS	WEB SITE ADDRESS	COMMENTS
Ace	01670 528204	info@ace.co.uk	www.co.uk	POP:UK coverage. Free web space
BT Internet	0800 800001	Info@bt.net	www.btinternet.com	POP:UK coverage. Free web space
Cable Internet	0500 541542	Info@cableinet.co.uk	www.cableinet.co.uk	POP: 36 UK towns and cities. PPP, free web space, multiple e-mail addresses
Demon Internet	0181-371 1234	Sales@demont.net	www.demon.net	POP:UK coverage. PPP, POP3 e-mail, FTP archive, free demo available
Easynet	0171-209 0990	Admin@easy.net.co.uk	www.easynet.co.uk	POP:UK coverage. Free web space.
EdNet	0131-466 7003	Info@ednet.co.uk	www.ednet.co.uk	POP: Edinburgh. PPP, POP3 e-mail, web and FTP space.
Freeserve	0906 553 5600		www.freeserve.net	POP:Hemel Hempstead. Free web space and Unlimited e-mail addresses.
Global Internet	0181-957 1005	Info@globalnet.co.uk	www.globalnet.co.uk	POP:UK coverage. PPP and web space available.
Hiway	01635 550660	Info@inform.hiway.co.uk	www.hiway.co.uk	POP:UK coverage. POP3 e-mail, free web space, FTP archive and space.
IBM Global Network	0800 973000	Internet_europe@vnet.ibm.com	Regsvr01.fl.us.ibm.net/cgi-bin/fees?ISO=gb	POP: Bristol, Edinburgh, Glasgow, Leeds, London, Manchester, Nottingham, Portsmouth, and Warwick. Various subscriptions option available.
KENTnet Internet Services	01580 890089	Sales@kentnet.co.uk	www.kentnet.co.uk	POP:Ashford, Hastings, Heathfield, Maidstone, Rye, Staplehurst, Tunbridge Wells. Free web space, FTP archive, domain registration, and conferencing.
London Web	0181-349 4500	Contact@londonweb.net	www.londonweb.net	POP:London. PPP, FTP and web space.
MANNET	01624 623841	Postmaster@mcb.net	www.mcb.net/mannet	POP:Isle of Man. PPP, FTP and web space available.
NetDirect Internet	0171-732 3000	Info@indirect.co.uk	www.indirect.co.uk	POP:London. PPP, FTP and web space, domain registration.
Oxford Community Internet	01865 856000	Info@community.co.uk	www.community.co.uk	POP:UK coverage. PPP, POP3 e-mail, web space.
Paradise Internet Network Services	01256 414863	Sales@pins.co.uk	www.pins.co.uk	POP:Basingstoke. PPP and web space available.
Rednet	01494 513333	Info@rednet.co.uk	www.rednet.co.uk	POP: UK coverage. PPP, free web space, POP3 e-mail.
Spud's Xanadu	01268 515441	Sweh@spuddy.mew.co.uk	www.spuddy.org	POP: Canvey Island. Free service, PPP, POP3 e-mail.
Taynet	01382 561296	Admin@taynet.co.uk	www.taynet.co.uk	POP: Dundee. PPP, POP3 e-mail, web space.
U-NET	01925 484444	Hi@u-net.com	www.u.net.com	POP: UK coverage. PPP, POP3 e-mail, web space.
Voss Net	01753 737800	Staff@vossnet.co.uk	www.vossnet.co.uk	POP: London, Slough. PPP, 7-day free trial.
Wave rider Internet	01564 795888	Info@waverider.co.uk	www.waverider.co.uk	POP: Birmingham. PPP, free web space, FTP archive.
Zetnet Services	01595 696667	Info@zetnet.co.uk	www.zetnet.co.uk	POP: UK coverage. Free web space, free trial.

Here is a list of countries, their country codes and whether or not they have Internet connection, e-mail-only connection or neither. For those countries that have Internet connection these are the two letters that you can expect to find at the end of World Wide Web domain names.

table A1 **The following countries have Internet connection**

COUNTRY CODE	COUNTRY	COUNTRY CODE	COUNTRY
AL	Albania	KW	Kuwait
DZ	Algeria	KG	Kyrgyz Republic
AD	Andorra	LV	Latvia
AQ	Antarctica	LB	Lebanon
AG	Antigua and Barbuda	LI	Liechtenstein
AR	Argentina	LT	Lithuania
AM	Armenia	LU	Luxembourg
AW	Aruba	MO	Macau (Ao-Me'n)
AU	Australia	MK	Macedonia
AT	Austria	MG	Madagascar
AZ	Azerbaijan	MY	Malaysia
BH	Bahrain	MT	Malta
BB	Barbados	MU	Mauritius
BY	Belarus	MX	Mexico
BE	Belgium	MD	Moldova
BZ	Belize	MC	Monaco
BI	Benin	MN	Mongolia
BM	Bermuda	MA	Morocco
BO	Bolivia	MZ	Mozambique
BR	Brazil	NA	Namibia
BN	Brunei Darussalam	NP	Nepal
BG	Bulgaria	NL	Netherlands
CA	Canada	NZ	New Zealand
KY	Cayman Islands	NI	Nicaragua
CF	Central African Republic	NO	Norway
CL	Chile	PK	Pakistan
CN	China	PA	Panama
CO	Colombia	PY	Paraguay
CR	Costa Rica	PE	Peru
HR	Croatia	PH	Philippines
CY	Cyprus	PL	Poland
CZ	Czech Republic	PT	Portugal
DK	Denmark	PR	Puerto Rico
DJ	Djibouti	RE	Reunion
DO	Dominican Republic	RO	Romania
EC	Ecuador	RU	Russian Federation
EG	Egypt	LC	Saint Lucia
SV	El Salvador	SM	San Marino
EE	Estonia	SA	Saudi Arabia
FO	Faroe Islands	SN	Senegal
FJ	Fiji	SG	Singapore
FI	Finland	SK	Slovakia
FR	France	SI	Slovenia
GE	Georgia	ZA	South Africa
DE	Germany	ES	Spain
GH	Ghana	LK	Sri Lanka
GI	Gibraltar	SR	Suriname
GR	Greece	SJ	Svalbarb and Jan Mayen Islands
GL	Greenland	SE	Sweden
GU	Guam	CH	Switzerland
GT	Guatemala	TW	Taiwan, Province Of China

table A1 *continued*

COUNTRY CODE	COUNTRY	COUNTRY CODE	COUNTRY
HN	Honduras	TH	Thailand
HK	Hong Kong	TT	Trinidad and Tobago
HU	Hungary	TN	Tunisia
IS	Iceland	TR	Turkey
IN	India	UG	Uganda
ID	Indonesia	UA	Ukraine
IR	Iran	AE	United Arab Emirates
IE	Ireland	GB	United Kingdom
IL	Israel	US	United States
IT	Italy	UY	Uruguay
JM	Jamaica	UZ	Uzbekistan
JP	Japan	VA	Vatican City State
JO	Jordan	VE	Venezuela
KZ	Kazakhstan	VI	Virgin Island (U.S.)
KE	Kenya	ZM	Zambia
KR	Korea (South)	ZW	Zimbabwe

table A2 **The following countries have e-mail-only connection**

COUNTRY CODE	COUNTRY	COUNTRY CODE	COUNTRY
AO	Angola	MW	Malawi
AI	Anguilla	ML	Mali
BS	Bahamas	MH	Marshall Islands
BD	Bangladesh	NR	Nauru
BA	Bosnia-Herzegovina	AN	Netherlands Antilles
BW	Botswana	NC	New Caledonia
BF	Burkina Faso (Formerly Upper Volta)	NE	Niger
KH	Cambodia	NG	Nigeria
CM	Cameroon	NU	Niue
TD	Chad	PG	Papua New Guinea
CK	Cook Islands	VC	Saint Vincent and the Grenadines
CI	Cote D'ivoire	WS	Samoa
CU	Cuba	SC	Seychelles
ER	Eritrea	SL	Sierra Leone
ET	Ethiopia	SB	Solomon Islands
GF	French Guiana	SD	Sudan
PF	French Polynesia	SZ	Swaziland
GM	Gambia	TJ	Tajikistan
GD	Grenada	TZ	Tanzania
GP	Guadeloupe	TG	Togo
GN	Guinea	TO	Tonga
GY	Guyana	TM	Turkmenistan
HT	Haiti	TV	Tuvalu
KI	Kiribati	VU	Vanuatu (Formerly New Hebrides)
LA	Laos	VN	Vietnam
LS	Lesotho	YU	Yugoslavia

table A3 **The following countries have no Internet or e-mail connection**

COUNTRY CODE	COUNTRY	COUNTRY CODE	COUNTRY
AF	Afghanistan	YT	Mayotte
AS	America Samoa	FM	Micronesia
BT	Bhutan	MS	Montserrat
BV	Bouvet Island	MM	Myanmar
IO	British Indian Ocean Territory	NF	Norfolk Island
BI	Burundi	MP	Northern Maiana Island
CV	Cape Verde	OM	Oman
CX	Christmas Island (Indian Ocean)	PW	Palau
CC	Cocos (Keeling) Islands	PN	Pitcairn
KM	Comoros	QA	Qatar
CG	Congo	RW	Rwanda
DM	Dominica	SH	Saint Helena
TP	East Timor	KN	Saint Kitts and Nevis
GQ	Equatorial Guinea	PM	Saint Pierre and Miquelon
FK	Falkland Islands (Malvinas)	ST	Sao Tome and Principe
TF	French Southern Territories	SO	Somalia
GA	Gabon	SY	Syria
GW	Guinea-Bissau	TK	Tokelau
HM	Heard and Mcdonald Islands	TC	Turks and Caicos Islands
IQ	Iraq	UM	United States minor Outlying Islands
KP	Korea(North)	VG	Virgin Islands (British)
LR	Liberia	WF	Wallis and Futuna Islands
LY	Libyan Arab Jamahiriya	EH	Western Sahara
MV	Maldives	YE	Yemen
MQ	Martinique	ZR	Zaire
MR	Mauritania		

The list above has been adapted from Landweber (1996).[24]
Copyright 1996 Lawrence H. Landweber and the Internet Society. Unlimited permission to copy or use is hereby granted subject to inclusion of this copyright notice.

appendix 4   troubleshooting error messages

Unfortunately, there will be times when you try to visit a web site and instead you receive strange error messages. There is no point getting too worked-up about it. Just accept them as part of the magic of the Net. Here are some of the most common NetScape Navigator error messages, with suggested actions.

ERROR MESSAGE	MEANING
400- Bad request	It may be that you have not typed the URL correctly. ▶ Check the URL for errors, such as upper or lowercase letters, colons, forward slashes.
401- Unauthorised	You're are attempting to enter a forbidden site, or you've entered an incorrect password. ▶ If you do have access, try the site again, ensuring that you type your password correctly.
403- Forbidden	If you are not entitled to access a site or a certain document, then there isn't a lot you can do other than trying again at a later date.
404- Not found	It is most likely that you have typed the address incorrectly. It is also possible that the page has moved or is no longer available. ▶ Try typing the address again.
503- Service unavailable	The web site may be down for a variety of reasons. ▶ Try the site again at a later time or date.
File contains no data	It is possible that the document is being updated just as you tried to access it. ▶ Try again later.
Host unavailable	You are probably trying to access a site that is down for maintenance. ▶ Try again later.
Connection refused by host	You are trying to access a secure document without proper authority. ▶ If you think you have the right to that document, contact the site's Webmaster.
Unable to locate the server	You are using an incorrect URL, or the server does not exist anymore. ▶ If you are sure you got the correct URL, check that you are entering it correctly.
Network connection was refused by the server	The server is probably busy. ▶ Try again later.
Too many users	The site is very busy. ▶ Try again later.
Unable to locate host	You have probably lost connection or the website is down. ▶ Try clicking the Reload button on the toolbar

appendix 5   glossary of terms used in this book

Access code is a unique combination of characters, usually letters or numbers, used in communications as identification for gaining access to a computer. The access code is generally referred to as *Username* or user ID and *password*.

Account is a term used in computer science to describe a Record-keeping arrangement employed by a System Manager at a College or University, health organisation, and a Vendor of an online service. It helps Vendors to identify their subscribers, for example, for billing. System Managers of multi-user systems use it to identify their users for administration and security purposes. A personal computing account is rather like your bank account; this has a Password that 'only' you know, together with an account name (*Username*) that identifies you.

Address (or Location) box is the box where you type your favourite web site addresses. In Internet Explorer this box is labelled 'Address', whereas in NetScape Navigator it is labelled 'Location'.

Anonymous FTP Some FTP sites are called Anonymous because the system does not need to find out who you are before letting you in. You can log in to these sites by entering the word *Anonymous* for *Username* and for *password* you enter your e-mail address or simply type the word *guess*.

Archie is an older system that was and can still be used to quickly find files that are located on the FTP sites.

Archie servers are located around the *Internet*. It can help you find the exact location of the files you are looking for literally in seconds. These servers keep track of all the *anonymous FTP* public files on the Internet by searching the public directories of the FTP hosts on a regular basis and maintaining a list of all files.

Articles see posting.

Bandwidth is a general term for the amount of information that can be transferred over an Internet connection.

Bibliography is a list of background reading carried out for assigments but not cited as direct reference in the body of an essay/academic paper.

Bounce means to return undeliverable. If you mail a message to a bad address, it bounces back to your mailbox. Conversely, if your e-mail address is erroneous, when people attempt to reply to your message it bounces back to their mailbox.

Browser is a computer program that enables you to *view web pages* on the *Internet*. Although NetScape browser is a very popular program, its main competitor is Microsoft Internet Explorer. The main advantage of this application is that Microsoft gives it away for free, while NetScape is a commercial software package. There are things that NetScape can do and Internet Explorer can't, and vice versa, but in general they are equally powerful.

Cookies are small text-files that some *web sites* store on your computer so that they know who you are next time you visit.

Database can be described as a sophisticated electronic filing cabinet capable of storing and sorting large amounts of data in an organised manner. The data can be accessed quickly.

Desktop is a computer that is kept on top of a desk or any suitable hard work surface.

Dot Matrix is a fairly basic, but flexible printer. It can produce text or graphics in the form of a matrix of small dots, with each character formed by a series of pins striking a ribbon. They are generally used for jobs where the quality of the printing is not crucial.

Download is to copy files (of any type) to your own computer from some other computer. The opposite term is to *upload*.

Electronic mail or **e-mail**, is essentially a text system that allows messages to be passed from one user to reach another user who is connected to the *Internet* or a computer network.

FTP stands for File Transfer Protocol. It is a method of transferring files from one computer to another over the Net.

Full-duplex A full-duplex card can record your voice while playing the incoming voice. This enables both of you to talk at the same time (ideal for discussions). With half-duplex you can either talk or listen, but not both.

Gateway A program or device that acts as a kind of translator between two networks that wouldn't otherwise be able to communicate with each other.

Gopher is an older system that lets you find text information by using menus.

Hacker is a term normally used to describe a skilled programmer who invades systems and ferrets out information on individual computer access codes through a process of trial and error.

Headers are the lines of text that appear at the beginning of every *Internet* mail message.

Homepage is a term used on the *Internet* to refer to the first page of a *web site*.

Hosts are computers that are directly connected to the *Internet*.

HTML Hypertext mark-up language: a code used in documents to indicate how information is to be displayed on the *World Wide Web*. HTML files are read by a *web browser* and it interprets codes about the format and size of text and where links to other files are to be placed.

Hypertext (hyperlink) is a system of clickable texts used on the web. These clickable texts serve as a cross reference to another part of the document (or an entirely different document).

IBM (Short for International Business Machines) is an American computer manufacturer, with headquarters in Armonk, New York. The company is a major supplier of information-processing products in the United States and around the world. Its products are used in a wide variety of industries, including business, government, science, defence, education, medicine, and space exploration.

Inbox is a term used to describe the box that stores all your incoming mail until it is read.

Inkjet printers can be described as the 'poor man's' laser printers. The inkjet printing system prints characters and graphics by firing ink drops at the paper from thin nozzles. These printers use a replaceable ink cartridge that contains both the print head and the ink.

Internet can be defined as a system that lets thousands of computers all over the world talk to each other.

Laser printers are fast, flexible and sophisticated. They produce high quality printing. They work on similar principles to a photocopier, using a photosensitive drum, and can produce between 4 and 20 pages per minute.

Laptop is a type of computer light enough for you to use whilst resting it on your lap and because it weighs around 9 to 12 pounds it can also be carried around.

Links are *hypertext*, identifiable by being underlined and a different colour from the ordinary text around it. Links can take you to other documents or other parts of the same document. On the web, links can appear as text or pictures.

List server program is a piece of software on a computer that reads the e-mail you send. For example, if you send an e-mail to subscribe to a list, it will automatically add your e-mail address to its list. For automatic lists, it is important that your e-mail request is constructed in a certain way.

Mailing list This term has two meanings: (a) a list of e-mail addresses to which you can send the same message without making endless copies of it, all with different addresses inserted and (b) a discussion group similar to newsgroups, but all the messages sent to the group are forwarded to its members by e-mail.

Modem is a device that converts the information on a computer into sound so that it can travel down the telephone line, and once it gets to the other end, the modem converts it back again into its original form.

News server is a computer (or program) dedicated to transferring the contents of newsgroups around the Net, and to and from your computer. This may be referred to as an NNTP server. These computers are maintained by companies, organisations and individuals, and can host thousands of *newsgroups*.

Newsgroup is a collection of messages posted by individuals to a *news server*.

Newsreader is the software program you use to access newsgroups, and to read, send, and reply to articles.

Online is a synonym for "connected". Anything connected to your computer and ready for action can be said to be online. In *Internet* terms it means that you have successfully dialled in to your service provider's computer and are now connected to the Net. The opposite term is *offline*.

Password is a secret code used to keep things private.

Posting When you send an e-mail message, the word 'sending' is quite good enough. When you send a message to a *newsgroup*, it isn't. Instead, for no adequately explained reason, the word *posting* is used. The word *article* is used to describe the message itself.

Public domain is material that, for whatever reason, is not protected by copyright law and can be used freely without permission. An example is a copyright that has expired.

RAM An acronym for Random Access Memory. It is a temporary storage space for information you are currently working on.

Reference list This can be defined as the bibliographical details of documents that support statements made in the main body of an essay/thesis.

Refresh rate is the rate the electrons scan the screen. Your computer measures this rate in hertz (Hz). The higher the rate, the better.

Search engines are indexes of WWW sites built automatically by a program called a spider, a robot, or a worm. These programs constantly scour the web and return with information about a page's location, titles and contents, which is then added to an index. For example, to search for a certain type of information, you just type in keywords and the search engine will display a list of sites containing these words. Search engines have the benefit of being up-to-date but the downside is that if, for example, you search for viral meningitis, the resulting list won't necessarily contain information about meningitis of the viral type – some may just be pages in which the words 'viral' and 'meningitis' both happen to appear. Directories don't have this problem because they list the subject of page rather than the words it contains, but the downside is that they won't always find the newest sites. Sites get listed in directories when their authors submit them for inclusion. See web directories.

Service Provider is a general term for a company that gives you access to the Internet by letting you dial in to its computer. This may be an Internet service provider (ISP) or an online service provider (IOP).

SLIP and **PPP** (SLIP is short for Serial Line Internet Protocol and PPP is short for Point-to-Point Protocol). They are *Internet* standards for transmitting Internet Protocol (IP) packets over serial lines (phone lines). Internet information is packaged into IP packets, a method for enclosing data into small, transmittable units (wrapped up on one end, unbundled on the other). A service provider might offer SLIP, PPP, or both. Your computer must use connection software (usually provided by the service provider) that matches the protocol of the server's connection software. PPP is a more recent and robust protocol than SLIP. So if you have a choice, select PPP.

Software Broadly speaking, it refers to the programs that provide the driving force of all computing systems. There are two types: operating systems software and applications software.

Tag is the name for *HTML* codes added to a plain text in a document. This transforms it into a web page with full formatting and links to other files and pages.

Telnet is a system that lets you connect from your computer to another across the *Internet* and use it as if you were directly connected to that computer. A slightly different version of Telnet, developed by *IBM*, is known as tn3270.

Thread is an ongoing topic of conversation is a *newsgroup* or *mailing list*. When someone posts a message with a new Subject line they're starting a new thread. Any replies to this message and replies to replies, and so on will have the same Subject line and continue the thread.

U-NET limited is one of several *Internet Service Providers* (ISP). It is a service that is aimed solely at Windows users. For a list of other ISPs refer to <u>Appendix 2</u>.

URL (pronounced 'earl') is the unique 'address' of a file on the Internet.

Usenet news system is a world wide bulletin board system which allows you to take part in discussions on a wide range of topics and is the main public discussion space on the Net.

Username is a unique name you are assigned by a service that enables you to connect to it and identify yourself, demonstrating that you are entitled to access it.

Web directories are hand-built lists of pages sorted into categories. Although you can search directories using a keyword search, it's often as easy to click on a category, and then click your way through the ever-more-specific subdirectories until you find the subject you're interested in. See search engines.

Web page is a single document that can be found on the web. It can be any length, like a document in a word processor. Pages can contain text, graphics, sound and video-clips, together with clever effects and controls. (A group of web pages is a *web site*. The first page of a web site is often called the *homepage*.)

Web site is a term loosely used to refer to a group of pages on the web. A site could be a single page or several complex pages belonging to a University, College, NHS Trust or a Nurse Therapist.

Windows can be described as a collection of programs, or suite of programs, written for personal computers and published by Microsoft. It is sometimes referred to as a GUI (graphical user interface). There are three common versions around: Windows 3.1, Windows95 and Windows98. The Third one is the most recent and most sophisticated.

World Wide Web (Also know as WWW, W3 or simply the web). A distributed information service based around *online hypertext* documents accessed using the *web browser* like NetScape or Microsoft Internet Explorer. The system was developed by an Englishman, Tim Berners-Lee, at CERN, European centre for research into particle physics, in Switzerland.

references (vancouver system citation — see section 9.3.2)

1. Ballard, E. 'Getting to grips with it! – Is it worth the effort?' In: *Newsletter* 2(1), 1996 Oct [WWW]. Available from: <http://www.shef.ac.uk/uni/projects/ctinm/ newslet/archives/balla.htm> [Accessed: 15 January 1998].

2. Howson, N. 'What use is the Internet to Nurses'. In: *CTI Newsletter* 3(1) 1997 Oct: pp 6–7.

3. Hoyler, A. *Internet UK in easy steps.* Warwickshire: Computer Step, 1997.

4. Gallagher, J. 'Web search tools: An Educational Evaluation'. 1995. [Online]. Available from: <http://cnet.unb.ca/clrn/nb/l/pages/enfe/evaluate/>

5. Leighton, H.V. 'Performance of four World Wide Web (WWW) index services: Infoseek, Lycos, Web-crawler and WWW Worm'. 1995. [Online]. Available from: <http://www.winona.msus.edu/services-f/library-f/ webind.htm>

6. Notess, G.R. 'Searching the World-Wide-Web: Lycos, WebCrawler and more' *Online Currents*, 1995 July/August: 48–53.

7. Stanley, T. 'Searching the World Wide Web with Lycos and InfoSeek'. 1995. [Online]. Available from: <http://www.leeds.ac.uk/ucs/docs/fur14/fur14.html>

8. Winship, I. 'World Wide Web searching tools – an evaluation'. 1995. [Online]. Available from: <http://www.bubl.bath.ac.uk/BUBL/IWinship.html>

9. Wilson, K. 'A review of three search engines including Infoseek'. *Online Currents*, 10(4), 1995 May: 5–6.

10. Murray, P.J. (1998) 'Nurses talking on-line: Who's out there and what are they saying?' In: *Newsletter,* 2(3) 1997 June. [WWW]. Available from: <http://www.shef.ac.uk/uni/projects/ctinm/newslet/archives/nurses.htm> [Accessed 15 January 1998].

11. Levine, J., Young, M. L., Reinhold, A. *The Internet for Dummies – Quick Reference.* 3rd Edition. IDG Books Worldwide Inc. Forster City. 1997.

12. Arlene Rinaldi. *The Net: User Guidelines and Netiquette.* 1996. [WWW]. Available from: <http://www.fau.edu/rinaldi/net/user.html> [Accessed 15 January 1998].

13. Howson, N. 'ScHARRP-Eyed: What use is the Internet for Nurses? Keeping Current on the Net'. In: *CTI Newsletter* 1998 June 3(3): pp12–13.

14. Harmon, C. *Using the Internet Online Services and CD-ROMS for Writing Research and Term Papers.* New York: Neal-Schuman Publishers, Inc. 1996.

15. Tseng. G., Poulter, A., & Hion, D. (1996) *The Library and Information Professional's Guide To The Internet.* London: Library Association Publishing. 1996.

16. McKenzie, B. C. *Medicine and the Internet – Introducing online resources and terminology*. Oxford: Oxford University Press. 1995.

17. Newall.E. 'Feedback'. [Personal memo to Chellen.S.S]. 1999. Available from <ssc1@cant.ac.uk>. [Accessed: 24 March 1999].

18. Couchman, D. 'Research and the Internet'. In: *Writers' and Artists' year book 1999*. 92nd Edition. London: A & C Black. 1999.

19. Howe, J. 'Referencing the Internet'. In: *Nursing Standard*. 1998. Sept 23–29, *13*(1): 28.

20. Dwyer, M. 'A guide to the Harvard referencing system'. In: *British Journal of Nursing*. 1995, *4*(10): 599–602.

21. St. George's Library. 'Referencing: Harvard System'. [WWW]. Available from: <http://www.sghms.ac.uk/library/harefern.htm> [Accessed: 11 February 1999].

22. Li, X. & Crane, N.B. *Electronic Styles – A Handbook for citing electronic information*. Medford: Information Today, Inc. 1998.

23. British Telecommunications plc. *Home Highway*. London. 1998.

24. Landweber, L.H. 'The Internet'. 1996. [WWW]. Available from: <http://info.lut.ac.uk/departments/ed/research/internet/inetble2.html> [Accessed: 10 October 1999].

recommended further reading (harvard system citation – see section 9.3.2)

Anon (1996) 'Nurses' Guide to the Internet: purchasing a home computer system and getting connected'. In: *AORN Journal, 64*(1): 112–114.

Anthony, D. (1996) 'Connecting to the InterNet'. In: *Health Informatics, 2*(2): 78–80.

Bowers, L. (1997) 'Constructing international professional identity: what psychiatric nurses talk about on the Internet'. In: *International Journal of Nursing Studies, 34*(3): 208–212.

Dwyer, M. (1995) 'A guide to the Harvard referencing system'. In: *British Journal of Nursing, 4*(10): 599–602.

Fleck, E. (1999) 'Internet support for nurses and midwives'. In: *Professional Nurse, 14*(4): 280–282.

McKibbon, K. (1998) 'Searching for the best evidence. Part 2: Searching CINAHL, and Medline'. In: *Evidence-Based Nursing, 1*(4): 105–107.

Musker, M. (1997) 'Demystifying the Internet: a guide for nurses'. *Nursing standards, 12*(11): 153–157.

O'Hara, S. (1994) *10 Minute guide to buying a computer*. Indiana: Alpha books – Macmillan Computer Publishing.

Osbourne, J. (1997) 'Student nurses on the Internet'. In: *Nursing Standard, 11*(39): 49.

Pitcher, M. (1998) 'Internet sources on leg ulcer management'. In: *Journal of wound care, 7*(6): 313–316.

Riddlesperger, K. (1996) 'CINAHL: an exploratory analysis of the current status of nursing theory construction as reflected by the electronic domain'. In: *Journal of Advanced Nursing, 24*(3): 599.

Ryan, J.M. (1998) 'A & E nursing and the Internet'. In: *Accident and Emergency nursing, 6*(2): 106–109.

St. George's Library (no date). 'Referencing: Harvard System'. [WWW]. <http://www.sqhms.ac.uk/library/harefern.htm> [Accessed: 11 February 1999].

Tatlow, M.P. (1995) 'Flexible learning on the information superhighway: FLISH 95'. In: *Health Informatics, 1*(3): 132–136.

Van Lanker, M. (1996) 'A convert to the net'. In: *Nursing Standard,* 10(27): 23.

quality of public services 69

radiography 63
RAM 18, 19, 204
RCN Learning Disability Nurses
    Forum 59
RCN Nursing Standard Online 65
references 173, 175
    citation systems 68–9, 175–80
    databases 177, 179
    e-mail archives 178
    FTP sites 177
    Gopher 178
    Harvard/Vancouver styles 173–4,
        176–80
    Internet sources 174, 176–9
    mailing lists 179
    World Wide Web 176
refresh rate 19, 204
relevancy scores, search engines 81
research funding 65
resources, evaluation 172
    see also health information
Resources for Nurses and Families
    62
Rinaldi 312 114
ROT13 126
Royal College of Nursing 47, 59,
    65

scroll bars 37
SCSI hard disks 19
search
    combining terms 99–100
    databases 89–90
    limiting 93, 94–5
    printing finds 100
    refining 96–8
    results 75–6
    setting options 75
    strategy 6, 71, 75, 88–9
search engines 73
    choosing 78–9, 204
    e-mail addresses 106
    relevancy scores 81
    subscription 79
    using 79–81
    see also Lycos

self-registration 15
self-study 171
service provider 17, 194–5, 204
    see also Internet service provider;
        online service provider
session profile, FTP 148–9
shell accounts 22
signature, e-mail 107, 117
Simeon mail 101, 105–13
Site for Student Radiographers and
    Schools 63
sites of interest, bookmarking 85
SLIP 22, 204
smileys 115–16
software xiii, 6, 204
SOSIG 84–5
sound card 19
sources
    electronic, citations 175–80
    referencing 173–80
    see also information gateways;
        web sites
spamming 188–9
Spina Bifida and Hydrocephalus 48
statutory bodies, UK 44–9
stop button 37, 38, 43
Student Nurses' Network 56
subject headings 91
subject trees: see web directories
subscribers list, mailing lists 138
surfing the net 5, 6, 10
systems managers 13, 106

tags 157, 159, 204
talking 139–40
telephone charges 141
telephone line 20
Telnet 5, 10, 143, 152, 205
template file, web page 159
Terence Higgins Trust 44
terminal account 22
text, web page 34
thread 129, 205
time out message 40
tn3270 143
toolbar buttons 33, 37–8
track ball 19
tree display 96, 112

trolls 127, 188
Tseng, G. 132
tutorials 6, 171
Twins and Multiple Births
    Association 48

U-NET 25, 205
UK Central Council for Nurses 47
UK Directory of Medical and
    Healthcare Specialists 56
UK Internet service providers
    195–6
UK online services, service
    providers 194–5
UK statutory bodies, websites
    44–9
UK Vacancy Database 181
UKOLN 67, 90
universities, Internet 25, 26, 154,
    169
UNIX shell account 22
unsubscribing, mailing list 135–6
uploading 166, 202
URLs (Uniform Resource Locators)
    27, 34–5, 39, 205
    changing nature of 40
    entering 42–3
    FTP 145
    name extensions 35
    punctuation 35
    service types 35–6
US
    domain names 36
    Green Card lottery 188–9
    search tools 73
Usenet discussion groups: see
    newsgroups
Usenet news system 35, 121, 205
user agreement 13, 193–4
user ID 103, 200
user newsgroups, referencing 178
username
    access code 103
    choosing 24–5
    college computer account 13,
        103, 200, 205
    FTP 145–6
    hospital Trust 15

ISBN 0-415-22747-X

9 780415 227476

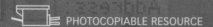

PHOTOCOPIABLE RESOURCE

'I have read this book and I love it. It is clear and informative. It is just right for any health care students, particularly those with little previous experience.'

Mooi Standing, Department of Nursing, Midwifery and Social Work, Canterbury Christ Church University College, Kent

'The units [in this book] are logical and systematic, offering a step-by-step guide to using the Internet. The content is nicely focused around health-related topics making this book more appealing to health-related students. It covers the topic area within health care exceptionally well.'

Rob McSherry, School of Health, University of Teeside

'I found this book most comprehensive and interesting. An invaluable resource for students particularly those that are fairly new to using the Internet to help with their studies…'

Keith Jones, Centre for Health Services Studies, The University of Kent at Canterbury and LASERNET

'This book has an easy reading level and an enthusiastic style. The layout is pleasing and leads the reader on…'

Nicola Eaton, School of Health Science, University of Wales, Swansea

There is a wealth of health information on the Internet. Today's students of health studies and all health care professionals must be able to use this valuable resource and extract from it what is most relevant and useful. In order for them to do this purposefully and skillfully, they need to have a thorough understanding of how the system works and have the ability to navigate their way around it with ease.

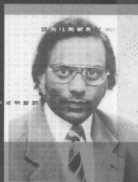

The Essential Guide to the Internet for Health Professionals is a superb photocopiable resource for lecturers and a self-instructional guide for students. It shows students:

↑ how to get online
↑ how to navigate the World Wide Web
↑ how to find health information on the Internet
↑ how to communicate with other health professionals
↑ how to access free health and medical resources
↑ how to publish on the web
↑ how to use online help with health studies assignments
↑ how to search for jobs

Each unit contains easy-to-follow activities and photocopiable worksheets. A special web site maintained by the author provides extra worksheets and updates to the information contained in this book, keeping readers abreast of important resources. Go to
http://www.routledge.com/routledge/feature/current/essential.html

Sydney S. Chellen is a Senior Lecturer in the Faculty of Nursing, Midwifery and Social Work, Canterbury Christ Church University College. He currently teaches Research and Information Technology to students on diploma, degree and other postgraduate programmes.

Health

11 New Fetter Lane,
London EC4P 4EE
29 West 35th Street,
New York NY 10001
Printed in Great Britain
www.routledge.com

DATE DUE

GAYLORD			PRINTED IN U.S.A.